The Easy Anti-Inflammatory Diet Recipes

50 Recipes for your Everyday Meals

Thomas Jollif

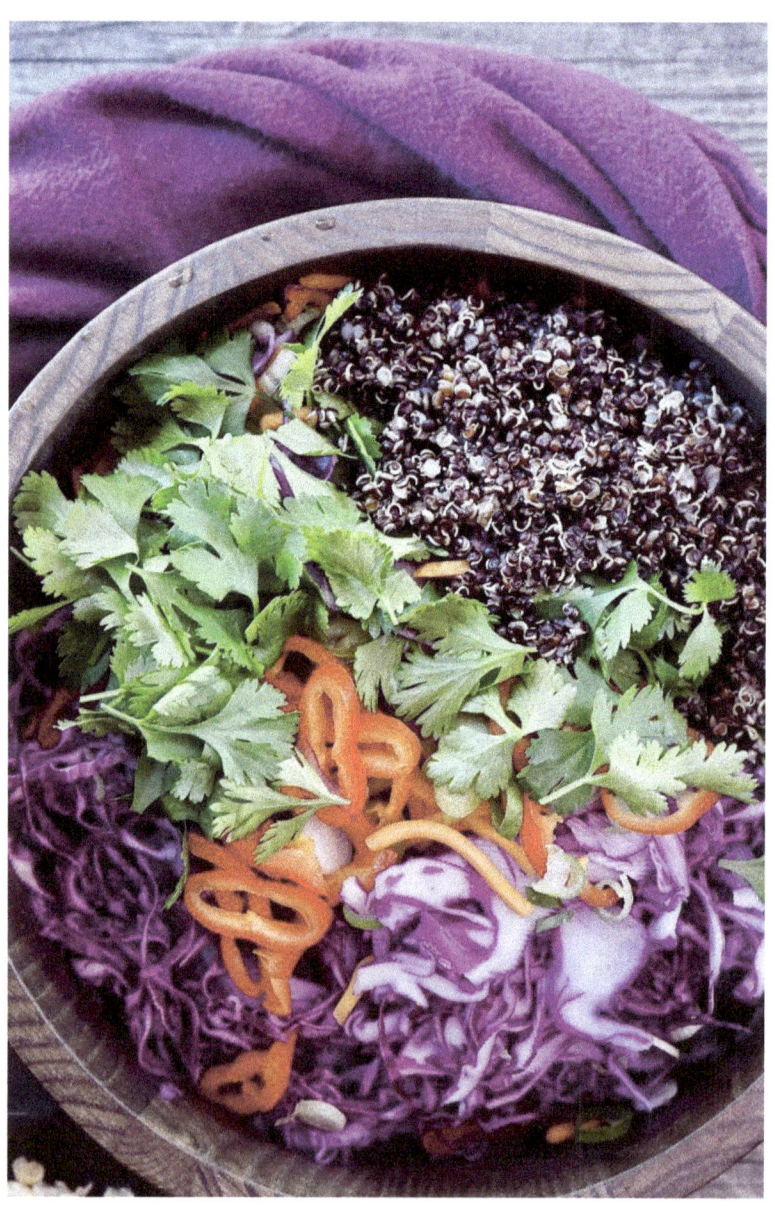

© copyright 2021 – all rights reserved.

the content contained within this book may not be reproduced, duplicated or transmitted without direct written permission from the author or the publisher.

under no circumstances will any blame or legal responsibility be held against the publisher, or author, for any damages, reparation, or monetary loss due to the information contained within this book. either directly or indirectly.

legal notice:

this book is copyright protected. this book is only for personal use. you cannot amend, distribute, sell, use, quote or paraphrase any part, or the content within this book, without the consent of the author or publisher.

disclaimer notice:

please note the information contained within this document is for educational and entertainment purposes only. all effort has been executed to present accurate, up to date, and reliable, complete information. no warranties of any kind are declared or implied. readers acknowledge that the author is not engaging in the rendering of legal, financial, medical or professional advice. the content within this book has been derived from various sources. please consult a licensed professional before attempting any techniques outlined in this book.

by reading this document, the reader agrees that under no circumstances is the author responsible for any losses, direct or indirect, which are incurred as a result of the use of information contained within this document, including, but not limited to, — errors, omissions, or inaccuracies.

Table of Contents

BREAKFASTS 7
   CARROT BREAD 7
   CARROT CAKE OVERNIGHT OATS 9
   CAULIFLOWER AND CHORIZO 10
   CHEDDAR AND CHIVE SOUFFLES 12
   CHEESY FLAX AND HEMP SEEDS MUFFINS 14
   CHERRY CHIA OATS 16
   CHICKEN MUFFINS 18
   CHOCO-BANANA OATS 20
   CILANTRO PANCAKES 22
   CINNAMON PANCAKES WITH COCONUT 24
   SMOOTHIES AND DRINKS 26
   BROCCOLI SMOOTHIE 26
   CARROT AND ORANGE TURMERIC DRINK 28
   CHERRY SMOOTHIE 30
   CHOCOLATE CHERRY SMOOTHIE 32
   CHOCOLATE LATTE WITH REISHI 34
   COOKED ICED TEA 36
   CUCUMBER KIWI GREEN SMOOTHIE 38
   CUCUMBER MELON SMOOTHIE 40

SIDES 42
   CUCUMBER YOGURT SALAD WITH MINT 42
   CURRY WHEATBERRY RICE 44
   FARRO SALAD WITH ARUGULA 46

    FETA CHEESE SALAD 48

    FRESH STRAWBERRY SALSA 49

SAUCES AND DRESSINGS 51

    CREAMY AVOCADO DRESSING... 51

    CREAMY HOMEMADE GREEK DRESSING 53

SNACKS 55

    BROWNIES AVOCADO 55

    BRUSCHETTA 58

    BRUSSELS SPROUT CHIPS 60

    BUTTERED BANANA CHICKPEA COOKIES 62

    CANDIED DATES 64

    CARROT STICKS WITH AVOCADO DIP 65

    CASHEW "HUMUS" 66

SOUPS AND STEWS 68

    CHICKEN CHILI BLANCO 68

    CHICKEN TORTILLA SOUP 70

    CHICKPEA CURRY SOUP 72

    CLEAR CLAM CHOWDER 74

    COCONUT CASHEW SOUP WITH BUTTERNUT SQUASH 76

    COCONUT CURRIED BAN-APPLE 78

    SOUP.. 78

    CREAM OF MUSHROOM SOUP 80

    CREAMY & CULTURE TOMATO SAUCE 82

    CREAMY BROCCOLI SOUP 84

    CREAMY CELERY AND CHICKEN BROTH 87

DESSERTS 89

BLUEBERRY TARTS *89*
CAFÉ-STYLE FUDGE *91*
CARAMELIZED PEARS *93*
CHOCO CHIA CHERRY CREAM *95*
CHOCOLATE BANANAS *96*
CHOCOLATE CHERRY CHIA PUDDING *97*
CHOCOLATE CHIP COOKIES *100*
CHOCOLATE CHIP QUINOA GRANOLA BARS *102*
CHOCOLATE COVERED STRAWBERRIES *104*
CHOCOLATE FUDGE BITES *106*

BREAKFASTS

Carrot Bread

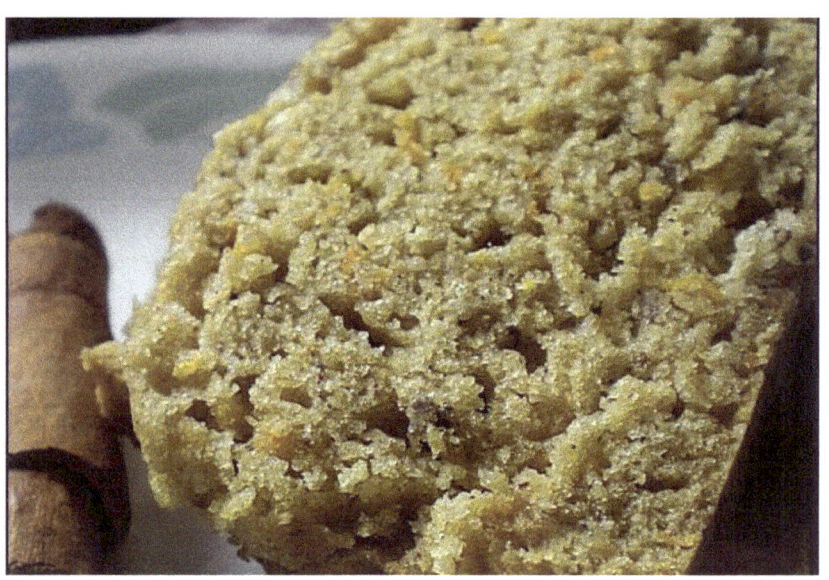

Time To Prepare: ten minutes
Time to Cook: 1 hour
Yield: Servings 8

Ingredients:

- ¼ cup sultanas
- ½-inch piece of fresh ginger, peeled and grated
- 1 tablespoon apple cider vinegar
- 1 tablespoon cumin seeds

- 1 teaspoon organic baking powder
- 2 cups almond meal
- 2 tablespoons macadamia nut oil
- 3 cups carrot, peeled and grated
- 3 organic eggs
- Salt, to taste

Directions:

1. Set the oven to 35 F, then line a loaf pan using parchment paper.
2. In a big container, put together the almond meal, baking powder, cumin seeds, and salt and mix.
3. In another container, put in eggs, nut oil, and vinegar and beat till well blended.
4. Place the egg mixture into the flour mixture and mix till well blended.
5. Fold in rest of the ingredients.
6. Put the mixture into prepared loaf pan equally.
7. Bake for approximately 1 hour.

Nutritional Info: Calories: 215 ‖ Total Fat: 17.1g ‖ Total Carbohydrates: 10.8g ‖ Fiber: 4.1g Sugars: 3.9g ‖ Protein: 7.6g

Carrot Cake Overnight Oats

Time To Prepare: five minutes + overnight
Time to Cook: 0 minutes
Yield: Servings 1

Ingredients:

- ½ cup Raisins
- 1 cup Coconut or almond milk
- 1 Large Carrot, peel, and shred
- 1 tbsp. Chia seeds
- 1 tsp. Cinnamon, ground
- 1 tsp. Vanilla
- 2 tbsp. Cream cheese, low fat, at room temperature
- 2 tbsp. Honey

Directions:

1. Mix together all of the listed ingredients and store them in a safe fridge container overnight.
2. Eat cold in the morning. If you choose to warm this, just microwave for a minute and stir thoroughly before eating.

Nutritional Info: Calories 340 ‖ 32 grams sugar ‖ 8 grams Protein ‖ 4 grams Fat ‖ 9 grams fiber ‖ 70 grams carbs

Cauliflower and Chorizo

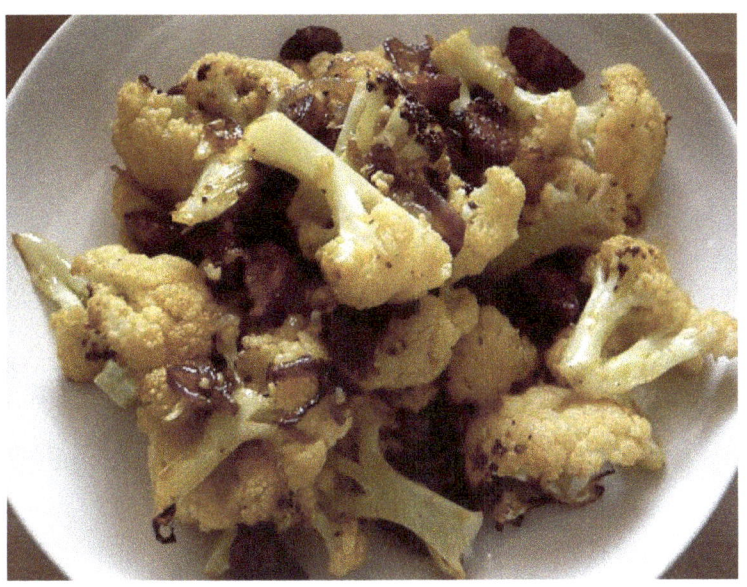

Time To Prepare: 55 minutes
Time to Cook: forty minutes
Yield: Servings 4

Ingredients:

- ½ teaspoon garlic powder
- 1 cauliflower head; florets separated
- 1 pound chorizo; chopped.
- 1 yellow onion; chopped.
- 12 ounces canned green chilies; chopped.
- 2 tablespoons green onions; chopped.
- 4 eggs; whisked

- Salt and black pepper to the taste.

Directions:

1. Heat a pan on moderate heat; put the chorizo and onion; stir and brown for a few minutes
2. Put in green chilies, stir, cook for a few minutes and take off the heat.
3. In your food processor, mix cauliflower with some salt and pepper and blend.
4. Move this to a container, put in eggs, salt, pepper, and garlic powder and whisk everything.
5. Put in chorizo mix as well, whisk again and move everything to a greased baking dish.
6. Bake using your oven at 375F then bake at least forty minutes.
7. Leave casserole to cool down for a few minutes, drizzle green onions on top, slice and serve

Nutritional Info: Calories: 350 ‖ Fat: 12 ‖ Fiber: 4 ‖ Carbohydrates: 6 ‖ Protein: 20

Cheddar and Chive Souffles

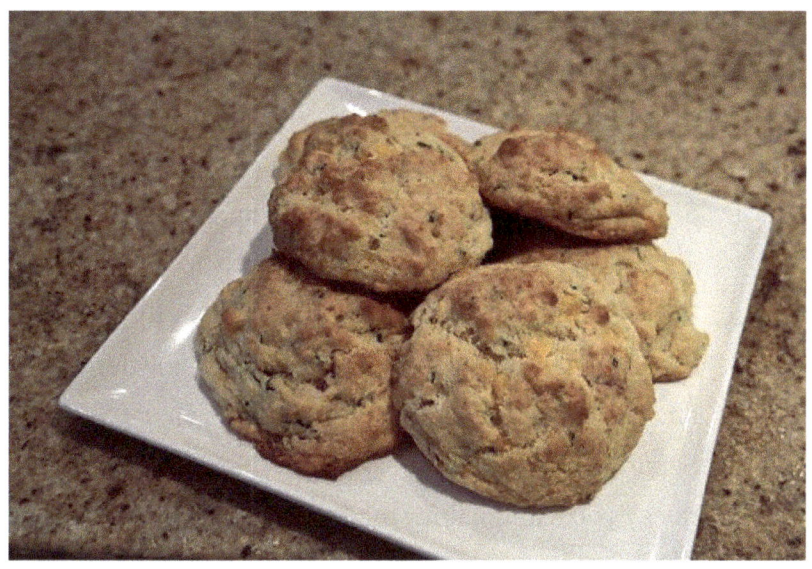

Time To Prepare: ten minutes
Time to Cook: twenty-five minutes
Yield: Servings 8

Ingredients:

- ¼ cup chopped chives
- ¼ tsp cayenne pepper
- ½ cup almond flour
- ½ cup baking powder
- ½ tsp cracked black pepper
- ½ tsp xanthan gum
- ¾ cup heavy cream

- 1 tsp ground mustard
- 1 tsp salt
- 2 cups shredded cheddar cheese
- 6 organic eggs, separated

Directions:
1. Switch on the oven, then set its temperature to 350°F and allow it to preheat.
2. Take a medium container, put in flour in it, put in rest of the ingredients, apart from for baking powder and eggs, and whisk until blended.
3. Separate egg yolks and egg whites between two bowls, put in egg yolks in the flour mixture and whisk until blended.
4. Put in baking powder into the egg whites and beat using an electric mixer until stiff peaks form and then stir egg whites into the flour mixture until thoroughly combined.
5. Split the batter uniformly between eight ramekins and then bake for about twenty-five minutes until done.
6. Serve straight away or store in your fridge until ready to eat.

Nutritional Info: Calories 288 ‖ Total Fat: 21g ‖ Carbs: 3g ‖ Protein: 14g

Cheesy Flax and Hemp Seeds Muffins

Time To Prepare: five minutes
Time to Cook: thirty minutes
Yield: Servings 2

Ingredients:

- ¼ cup almond meal
- ¼ cup cottage cheese, low-fat
- ¼ cup grated parmesan cheese
- ¼ cup raw hemp seeds
- ¼ cup scallion, cut thinly
- ¼ tsp baking powder
- 1 tbsp. olive oil
- 1/8 cup flax seeds meal
- 1/8 cup nutritional yeast flakes
- 3 organic eggs, beaten
- Salt, to taste

Directions:

1. Switch on the oven, then set it 360°F and allow it to preheat.
2. In the meantime, take two ramekins, grease them with oil, and set aside until required.

3. Take a medium container, put in flax seeds, hemp seeds, and almond meal, and then mix in salt and baking powder until combined.
4. Crack eggs in a different container, put in yeast, cottage cheese, and parmesan, stir thoroughly until blended, and then stir this mixture into the almond meal mixture until blended.
5. Fold in scallions, then spread the mixture between prepared ramekins and bake for thirty minutes until muffins are firm and the top is nicely golden brown.
6. When finished, take out the muffins from the ramekins and allow them to cool to room temperature on a wire rack.
7. For meal prepping, wrap each muffin using a paper towel and place in your fridge for maximum thirty-four days.
8. When ready to eat, reheat muffins in the microwave until hot and then serve.

Nutritional Info: Calories 179 ‖ Total Fat: 10.9g ‖ Carbs: 6.9g ‖ Protein: 15.4g ‖ Sugar: 2.3g ‖ Sodium: 311mg

Cherry Chia Oats

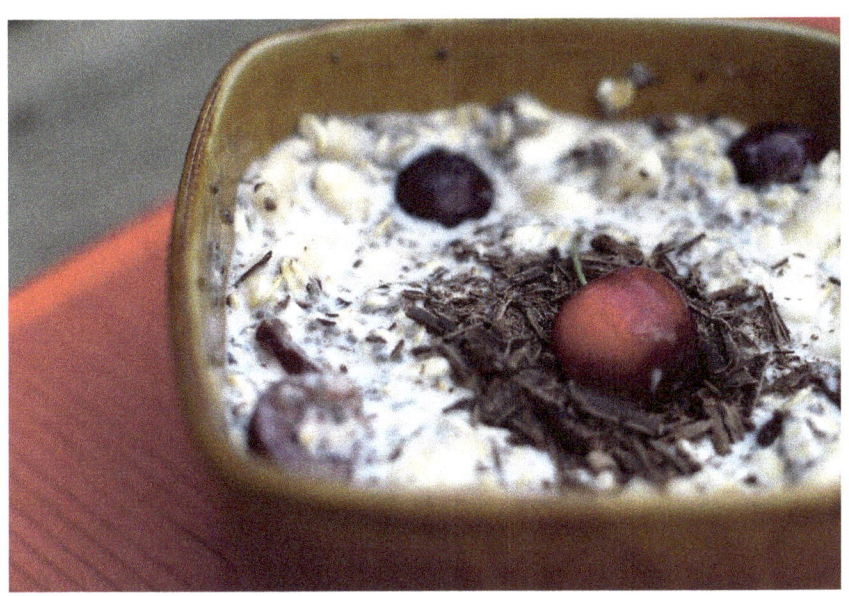

Time To Prepare: ten minutes
Time to Cook: twenty minutes
Yield: Servings 2

Ingredients:

- ¼ Cup Whole Milk Yogurt, Plain
- ¼ Teaspoon Vanilla Extract, Pure
- 1 ¼ Cup Almond Milk
- 1 Cup Quick Cook Oats
- 2 Tablespoons Almond Butter
- 2 Tablespoons Chia Seeds

- 8 Cherries, Fresh, Pitted & Halved

Directions:

1. Combine all the ingredients until they're blended well.
2. Seal in two jars and place in your fridge for twenty-five minutes before you serve.

Nutritional Info: Calories: 564 ‖ Protein: 22 Grams ‖ Fat: 32 Grams ‖ Carbohydrates: 27 Grams

Chicken Muffins

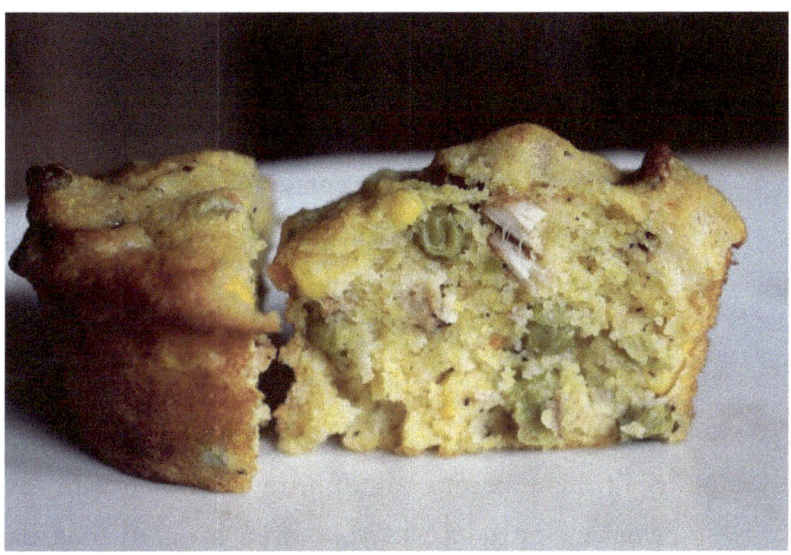

Time To Prepare: 1 hour ten minutes
Time to Cook: thirty minutes
Yield: Servings 3

Ingredients:
- ½ teaspoon garlic powder
- 2 tablespoons green onions; chopped.
- 3 tablespoons hot sauce mixed with 3 tablespoons melted coconut oil
- 3/4 pound chicken breast; boneless
- 6 eggs

- Salt and black pepper to the taste.

Directions:

1. Season chicken breast with pepper, salt, and garlic powder, place on a lined baking sheet, and bake in your oven at 425F for minimum twenty-five minutes.
2. Move chicken breast to a container, shred using a fork, and mix with half of the hot sauce and melted coconut oil.
3. Toss to coat and leave aside.
4. In a container, mix eggs with salt, pepper, green onions, and the remaining hot sauce mixed with oil and whisk very well.
5. Split this mix into a muffin tray, top each with shredded chicken, introduce in your oven at 350F then bake for minimum 30 minutes.
6. Serve your muffins hot.

Nutritional Info: Calories: 140 ‖ Fat: 8 ‖ Fiber: 1 ‖ Carbohydrates: 2 ‖ Protein: 13

Choco-Banana Oats

Time To Prepare: five minutes
Time to Cook: 8 minutes
Yield: Servings 2

Ingredients:

- ¼ tsp. almond extract
- ¼ tsp. Vanilla
- ¾ cup water
- 1/3 cup toasted walnuts, chopped
- 1/8 tsp. cinnamon
- 1/8 tsp. salt
- 2 cups almond milk
- 2 cups oats
- 2 ripe bananas, cut
- 2 tbsp. agave nectar
- 2 tbsp. cocoa powder, unsweetened
- 2 tbsp. vegan chocolate chips, semisweet

Directions:

1. In a big deep cooking pan, pour the almond milk, water, bananas, vanilla, and almond extract. Put in the salt, stir, and heat over high temperature.
2. Combine the oats in the pan together with the unsweetened cocoa powder, 1 tbsp. agave nectar and reduce the

temperature to moderate. Cook for 7-8 minutes, or until the oats are cooked to your preference. Stir regularly.
3. Scoop the cooked oats into serving bowls and decorate with the chopped walnuts, chocolate chips, and sprinkle with the remaining agave nectar.

Nutritional Info: Calories: 522 kcal ‖ Protein: 30.17 g ‖ Fat: 27.01 g ‖ Carbohydrates: 79.09 g

Cilantro Pancakes

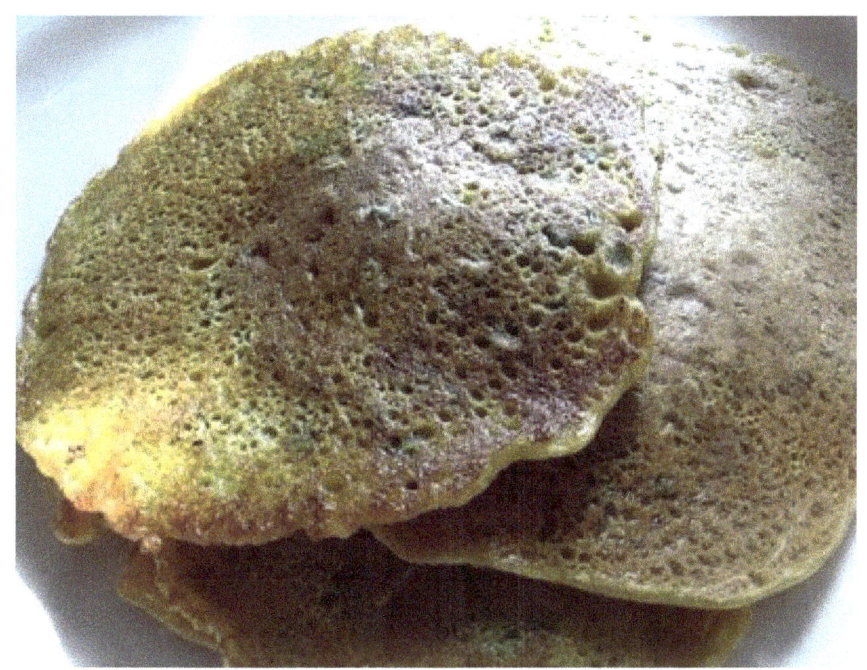

Time To Prepare: ten minutes
Time to Cook: 6-8 minutes
Yield: Servings 6

Ingredients:
- ¼ teaspoon ground turmeric
- ½ cup almond flour
- ½ cup fresh cilantro, chopped
- ½ cup tapioca flour
- ½ of red onion, chopped

- ½ teaspoon chili powder
- 1 (½-inch) fresh ginger piece, grated finely
- 1 cup full-Fat coconut milk
- 1 Serrano pepper, minced
- Freshly ground black pepper, to taste
- Oil, as required
- Salt, to taste

Directions:

1. In a big container, put together the flours and spices then mix.
2. Place the coconut milk and mix till well blended.
3. Fold within the onion, ginger, Serrano pepper, and cilantro.
4. Lightly, grease a sizable nonstick frying pan with oil and warmth on medium-low heat.
5. Put in about ¼ cup of mixture and tilt the pan to spread it uniformly inside the frying pan.
6. Cook for about four minutes from either side.
7. Repeat with all the rest of the mixture.
8. Serve together with your desired topping.

Nutritional Info: Calories: 331 ‖ Fat: 10g ‖ Carbohydrates: 37g ‖ Fiber: 6g ‖ Protein: 28g

Cinnamon Pancakes with Coconut

Time To Prepare: five minutes
Time to Cook: eighteen minutes
Yield: Servings 2

Ingredients:

- ¼ cup shredded coconut and more for decorationing
- ½ tbsp. erythritol
- ½ tbsp. olive oil
- 1 tbsp. almond flour
- 1 tsp cinnamon
- 1/8 tsp salt
- 2 organic eggs
- 2oz cream cheese
- 4 tbsp. stevia

Directions:

1. Crack eggs in a container, beat until fluffy and then beat in flour and cream cheese until the desired smoothness is achieved.
2. Put in rest of the ingredients and then stir until well blended.
3. Take a frying pan, place it on moderate heat, grease it with oil, then pour in half of the batter and cook for three to four

minutes per side until the pancake has cooked and nicely golden brown.
4. Move pancake to a plate and cook another pancake similarly by using the rest of the batter.
5. Drizzle coconut on top of cooked pancakes before you serve.

Nutritional Info: Calories 575 ‖ Total Fat: 51g ‖ Carbs: 3.5g ‖ Protein: 19g

Smoothies and Drinks

Broccoli Smoothie

Time To Prepare: five minutes
Time to Cook: 0 minutes
Yield: Servings 4

Ingredients:
- 1 ½ cups strawberries
- 1 ½ cups water
- 1 cup broccoli florets
- 1 cup chopped spinach
- 2 bananas, cut, frozen
- 2 cups frozen mango chunks
- 2 cups pineapple juice

Directions:
1. Combine all ingredients into a blender and blend until the desired smoothness is achieved.
2. Pour into 4 tall glasses before you serve.

Nutritional Info: Calories: 222 kcal ‖ Protein: 3.51 g ‖ Fat: 1.98 g ‖ Carbohydrates: 51.45 g

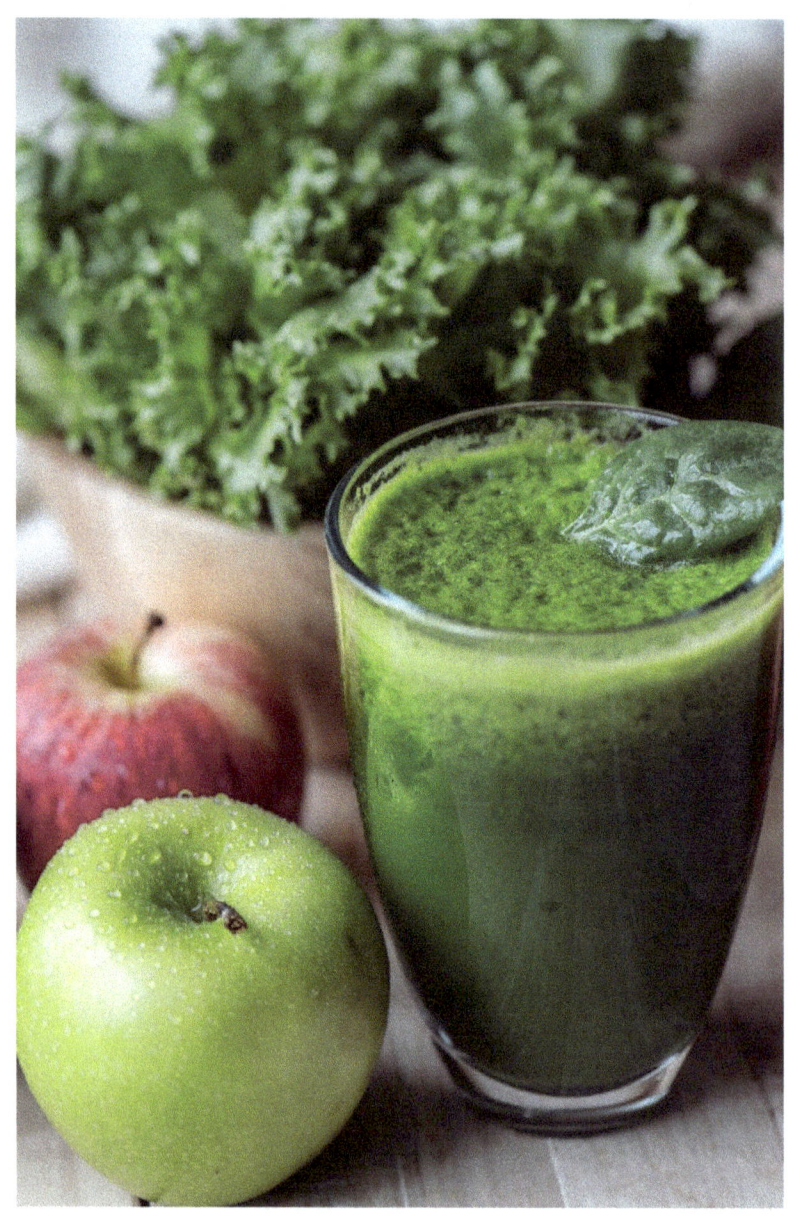

Carrot and Orange Turmeric Drink

Time To Prepare: five minutes
Time to Cook: 0 minutes
Yield: Servings 2

Ingredients:

- 1 cup orange juice
- 1 tbsp. lemon juice
- 1/2 inch ginger slice
- 1/4 tsp. turmeric powder
- 2 carrots, peeled, chopped
- 2 tbsp. sugar

Directions:

1. In a blender, put in orange juice, sugar, turmeric powder, carrots, and lemon juice.
2. Blend well.

Serve!

Nutritional Info: Calories: 153 kcal ‖ Protein: 4.47 g ‖ Fat: 3.3 g ‖ Carbohydrates: 27.02 g

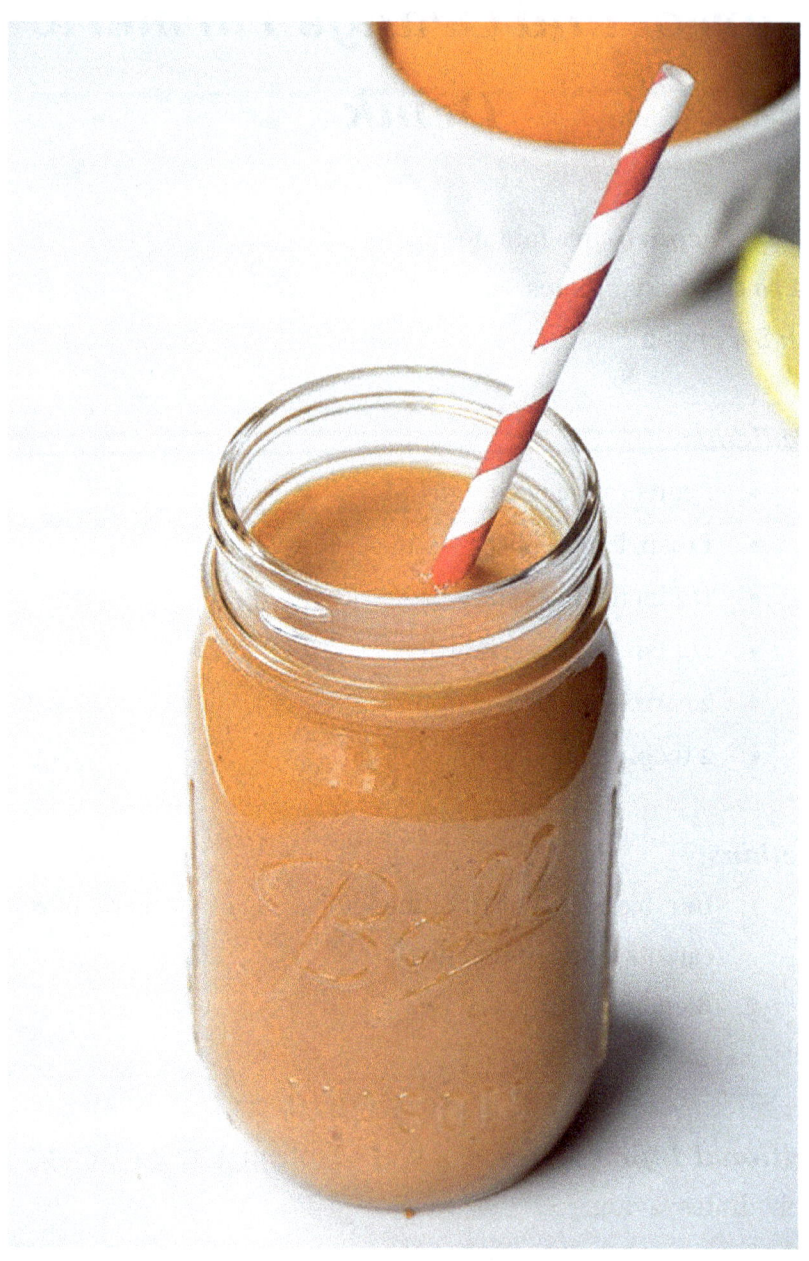

Cherry Smoothie

Time To Prepare: five minutes
Time to Cook: 0 minutes
Yield: Servings 4-6

Ingredients:

- 1 ½ cups vanilla Greek yogurt
- 2 bananas, cut
- 3 cups cherry juice
- 3 cups pitted, froze dark sweet cherries
- Fresh cherries, pitted
- Mint sprigs
- To decorate: Optional

Directions:

1. Combine all ingredients into a blender and blend until the desired smoothness is achieved.
2. Pour into 4 tall glasses.
3. Decorate using optional ingredients if using before you serve.

Nutritional Info: Calories: 114 kcal ‖ Protein: 2.36 g ‖ Fat: 1.88 g ‖ Carbohydrates: 23.49 g

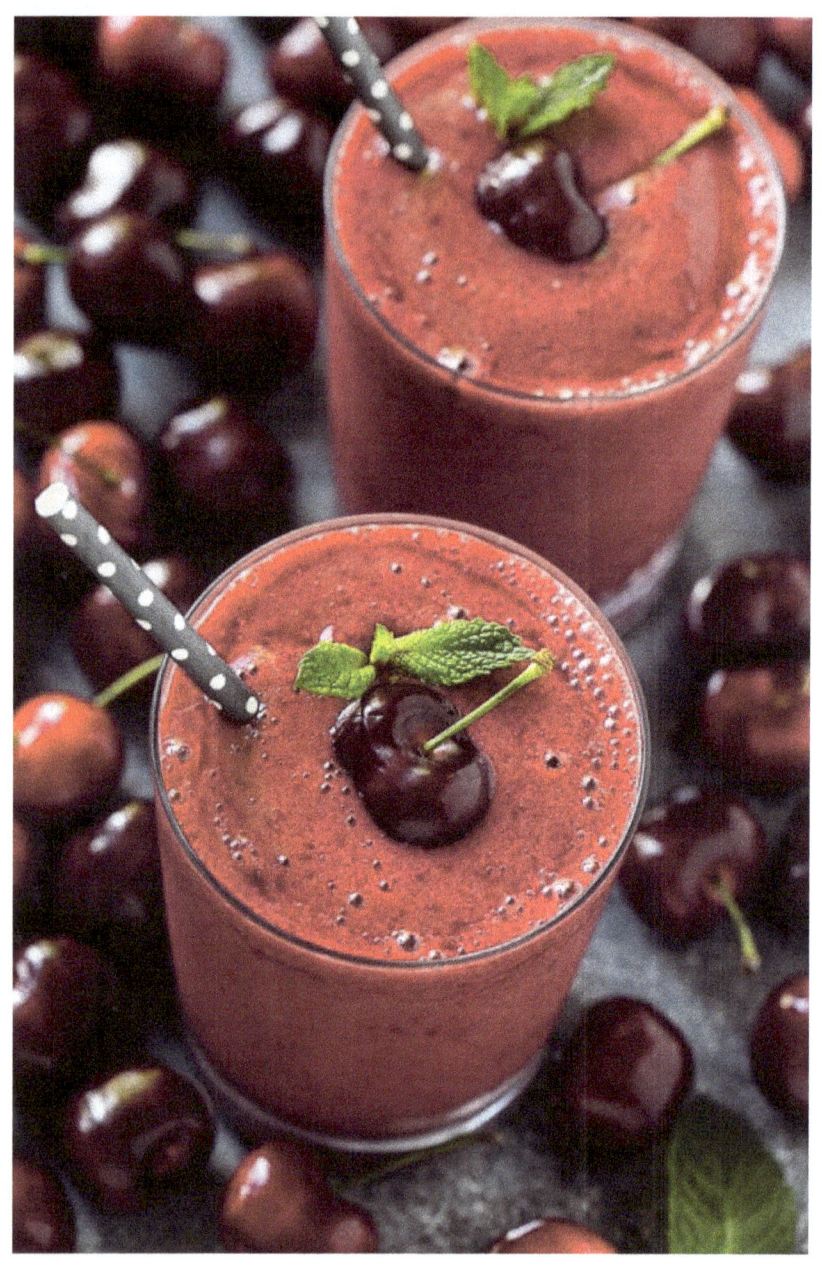

Chocolate Cherry Smoothie

Time To Prepare: five minutes

Time to Cook: 0 minutes

Yield: Servings 2

Ingredients:

- 2 cups almond milk, unsweetened
- 2 dates, pitted, chopped or 2 teaspoons pure maple syrup
- 2 scoops protein powder or 4 tablespoons almond butter (not necessary)
- 4 cups pitted, frozen cherries
- 4 tablespoons cocoa or cacao powder
- Cacao nibs
- Granola
- Hemp hearts
- To serve: Optional

Directions:

1. Combine all ingredients into a blender and blend until the desired smoothness is achieved.
2. Pour into 2 tall glasses and serve topped with optional ingredients.

Nutritional Info: Calories: 339 kcal ‖ Protein: 16.37 g ‖ Fat: 21.34 g ‖ Carbohydrates: 27.99 g

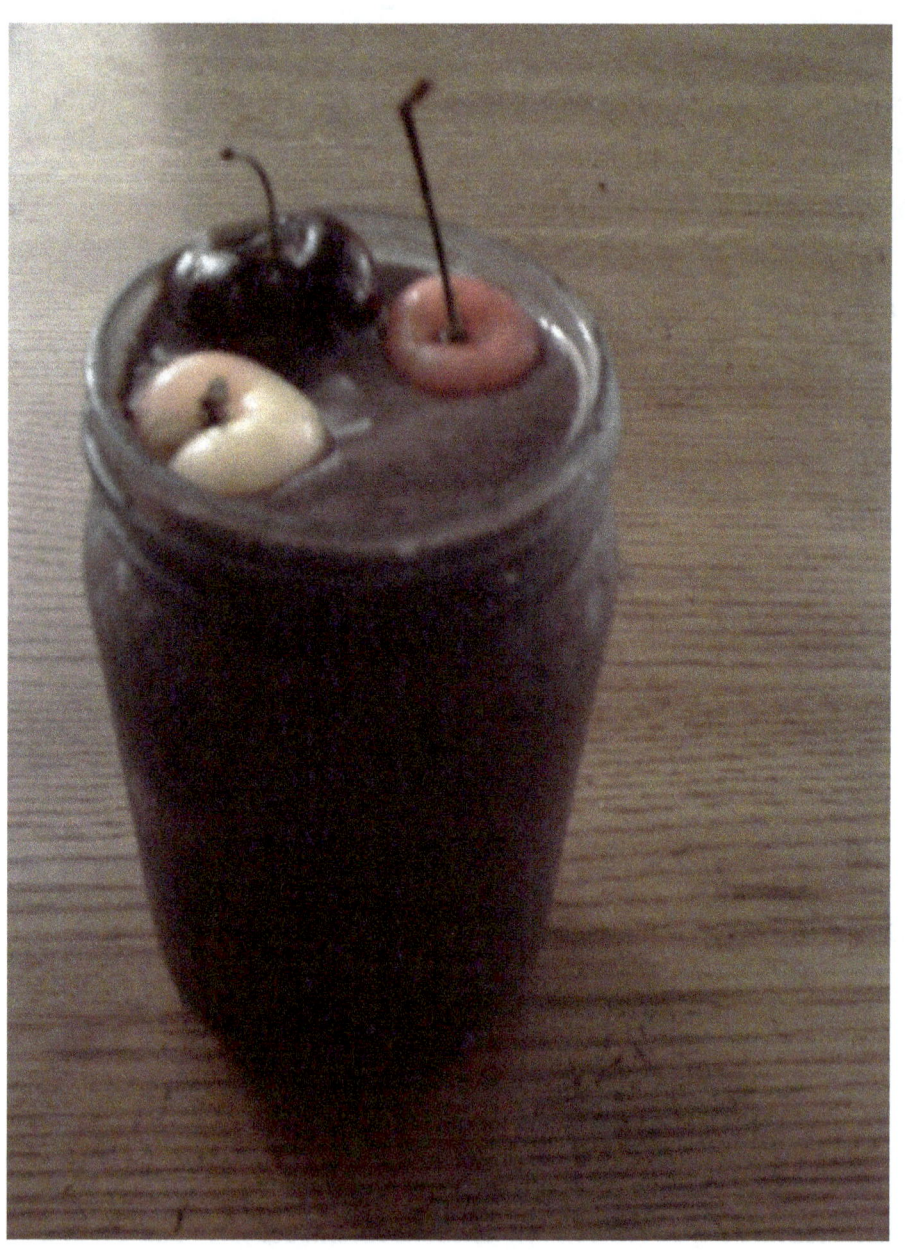

Chocolate Latte with Reishi

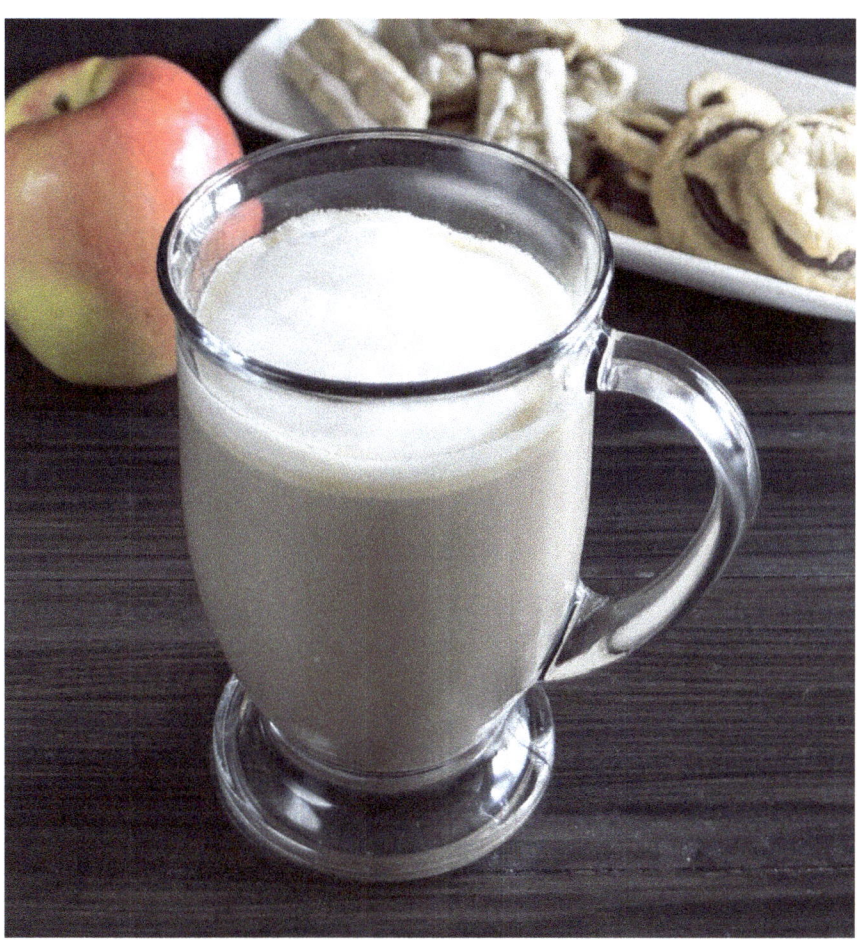

Time To Prepare: five minutes
Time to Cook: ten minutes
Yield: Servings 2

Ingredients:
- 1 teaspoon Reishi powder
- 2 tablespoons coconut butter
- 4 cups almond milk, unsweetened
- 4 teaspoons raw cacao powder
- A pinch ground cinnamon
- A pinch sea salt
- Sweetener of your choice

Directions:
1. Put in almond milk into a deep cooking pan. Put the deep cooking pan using low heat.
2. When the milk is warm and just starts to bubble, remove the heat. Move into a blender.
3. Put in the remaining ingredients and blend for 30 – 40 seconds or until the desired smoothness is achieved.
4. Pour into mugs before you serve.

Nutritional Info: Calories: 461 kcal ‖ Protein: 19.32 g ‖ Fat: 30.57 g ‖ Carbohydrates: 28.08 g

Cooked Iced Tea

Time To Prepare: two minutes
Time to Cook: 4 minutes
Yield: Servings 4

Ingredients:

- 2 tbsp. honey
- 4 regular tea bags
- 6 cups water

Directions:

1. Put in ingredients to the instant pot.
2. Secure the lid. Cook on HIGH pressure 4 minutes.
3. When done, depressurize naturally.
4. Allow to cool to room temperature. Serve over ice.

Nutritional Info: Calories: 22 ‖ Fat: 0g ‖ Carbohydrates: 6g ‖ Protein: 0g

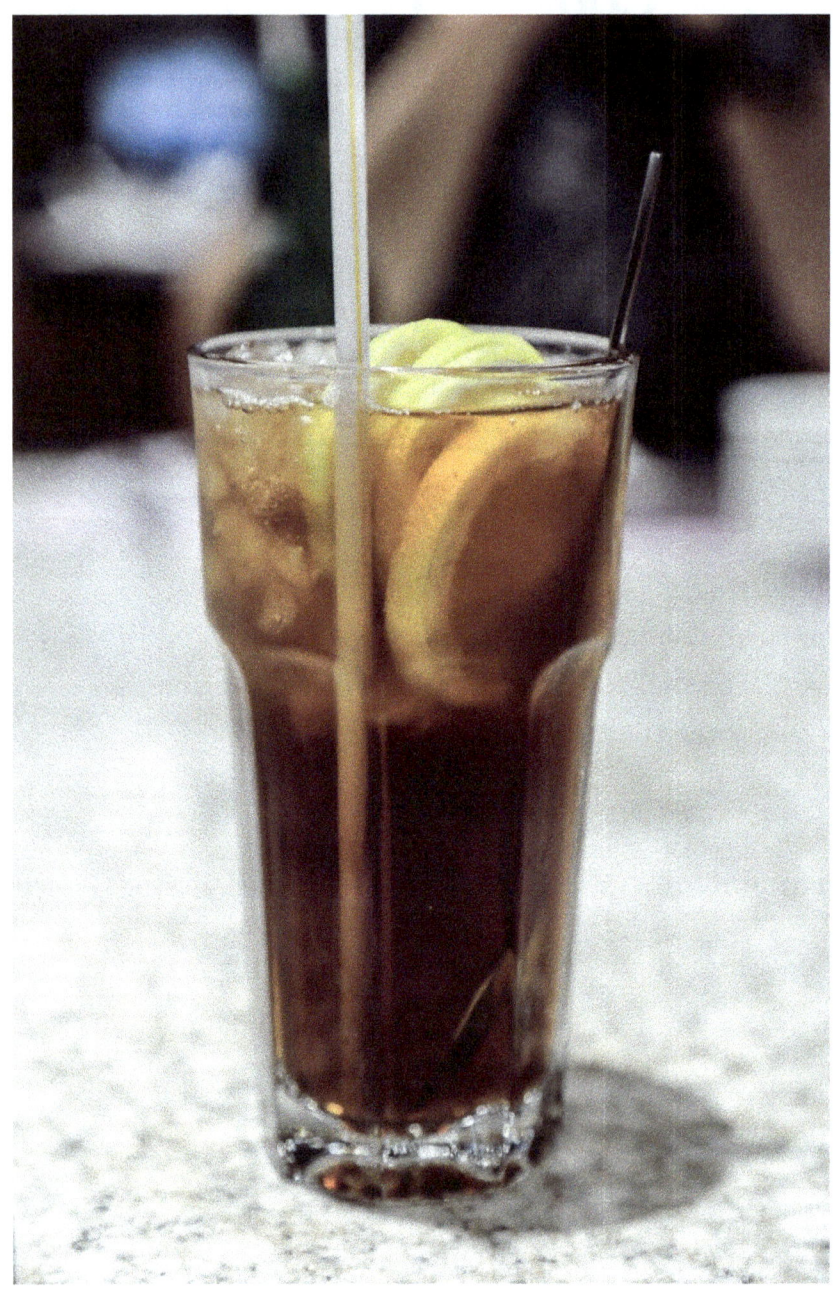

Cucumber Kiwi Green Smoothie

Time To Prepare: five minutes
Time to Cook: 0 minutes
Yield: Servings 2

Ingredients:

- ¼ cup of canned coconut milk
- 1 cup of coconut water
- 1 cup of seedless cucumber, chopped
- 2 ripe kiwi fruit
- 2 tbsps. of fresh chopped cilantro
- 6 to 8 ice cubes
- ice cubes

Directions:

1. Mix the smoothie ingredients in your high-speed blender.
2. Pulse the ingredients a few times to cut them up.
3. Combine the mixture on the highest speed setting for thirty to 60 seconds.
4. Pour into glasses and serve.

Nutritional Info: Calories: 140 kcal ‖ Protein: 5.1 g ‖ Fat: 10.52 g ‖ Carbohydrates: 7.4 g

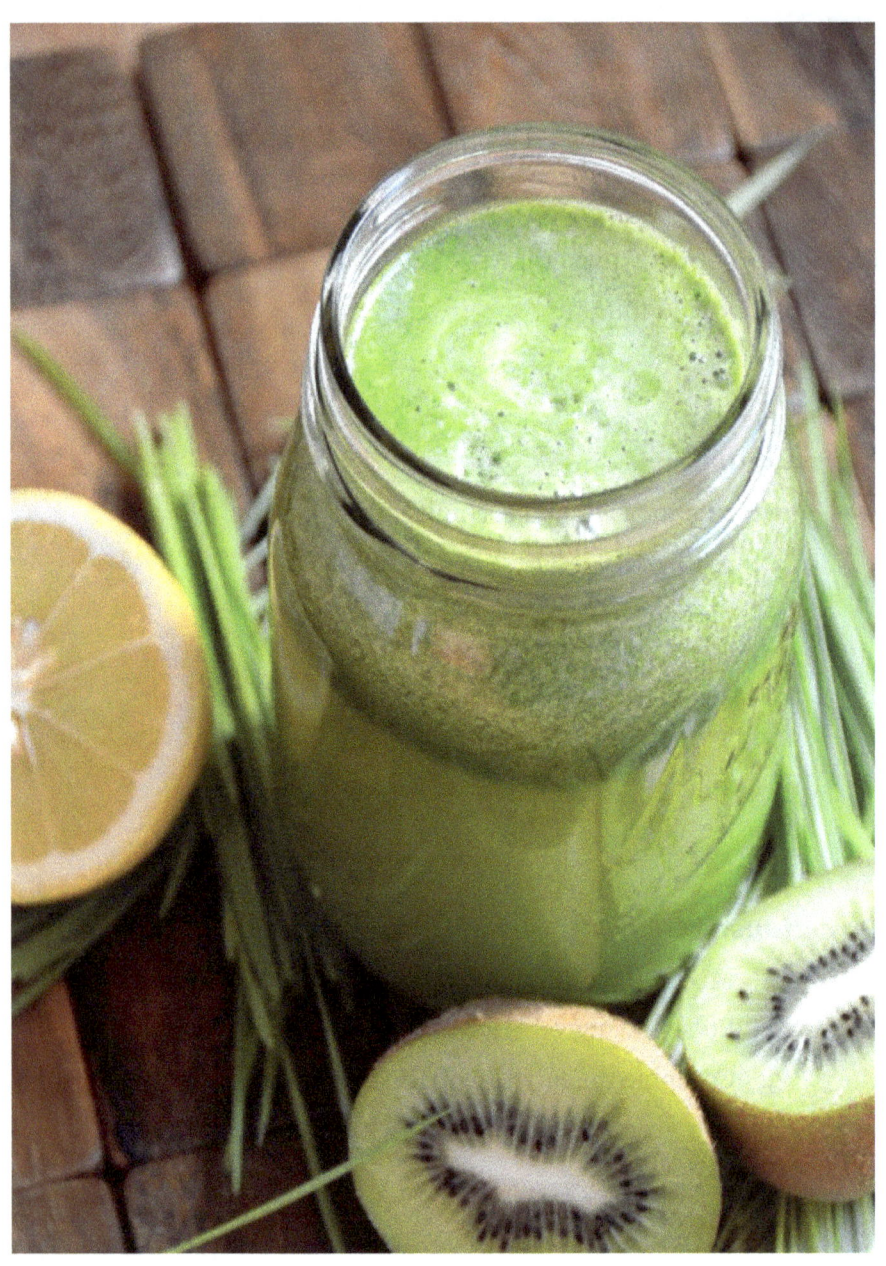

Cucumber Melon Smoothie

Time To Prepare: five minutes
Time to Cook: 0 minutes
Yield: Servings 2

Ingredients:

- 1 ½ cups of chopped honeydew
- 1 cup of chilled coconut water
- 1 cup of seedless cucumber, diced
- 2 tbsp. of fresh mint
- 6 to 8 ice cubes

Directions:

1. Mix the smoothie ingredients in your high-speed blender.
2. Pulse the ingredients a few times to cut them up.
3. Combine the mixture on the highest speed setting for thirty to 60 seconds.
4. Pour into glasses and serve.

Nutritional Info: Calories: 300 kcal ‖ Protein: 5.83 g ‖ Fat: 8.55 g ‖ Carbohydrates: 51.21 g

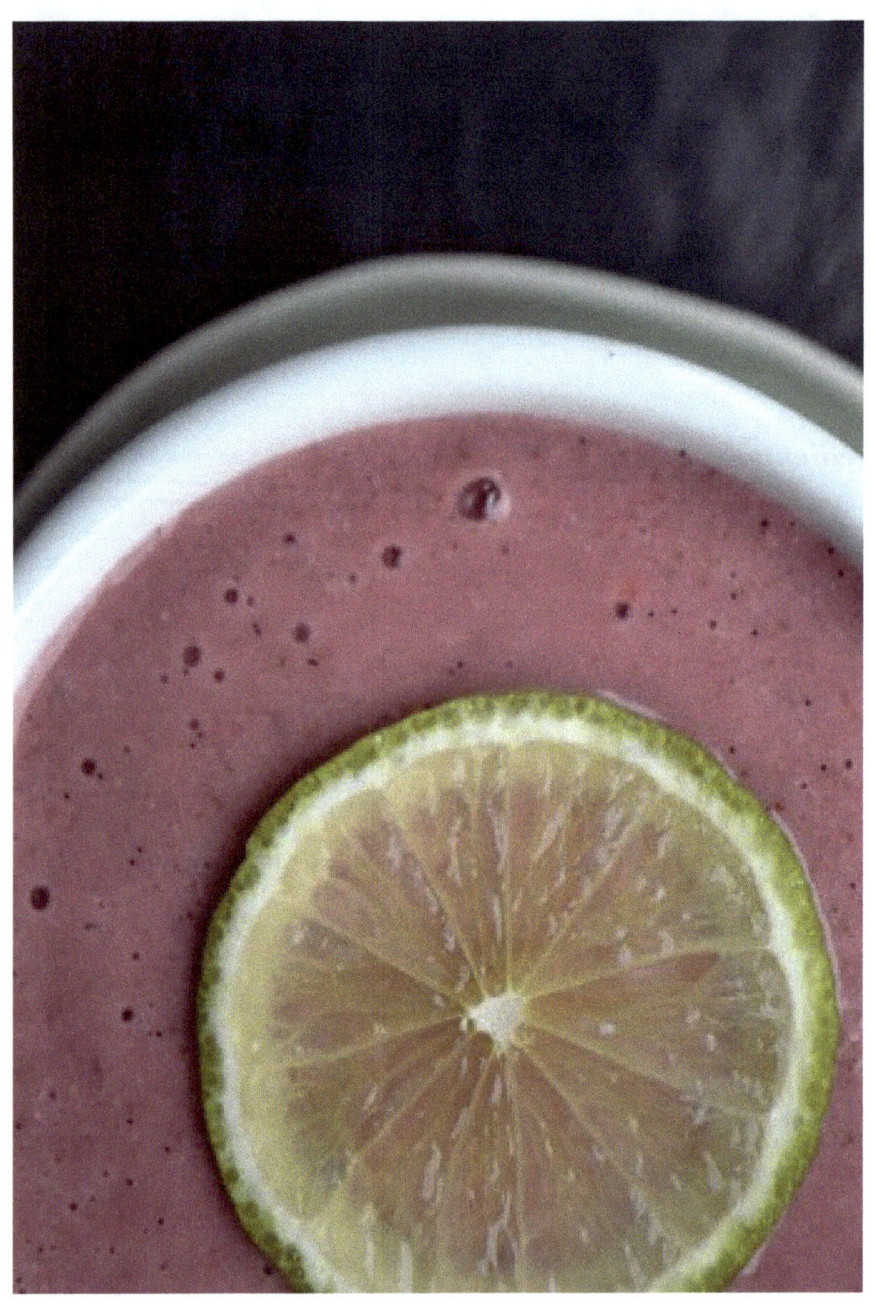

SIDES

Cucumber Yogurt Salad with Mint

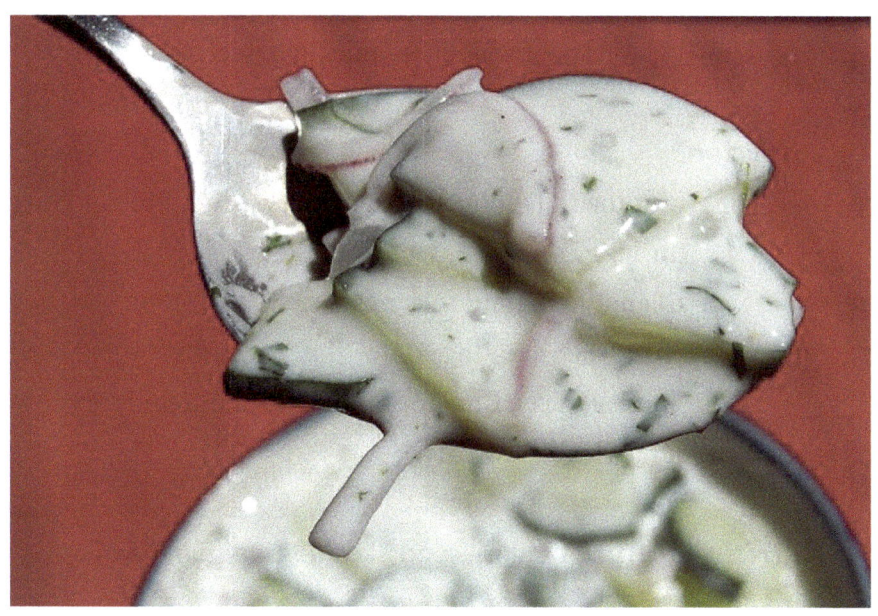

Time To Prepare: ten minutes
Time to Cook: 0 minutes
Yield: Servings 2

Ingredients:
- ¼ cup organic coconut milk
- ¼ cup organic mint leaves
- ¼ teaspoon pink Himalayan sea salt
- ½ cup chopped organic red onion
- 1 tablespoon extra virgin olive oil
- 1 tablespoon plain organic goat yogurt
- 1 teaspoon organic dill weed
- 2 chopped organic cucumbers
- 3 tablespoons fresh organic lime juice

Directions:
1. Cut the red onion, dill, cucumbers, and mint and mix them in a big container.
2. Blend them until they're smooth.
3. Top the dressing onto the cucumber salad and mix meticulously. Chill for minimum 1 hour and serve.
4. Enjoy!

Nutritional Info: ‖ Calories: 207 kcal ‖ Protein: 6.9 g ‖ Fat: 13.87 g ‖ Carbohydrates: 18.04 g

Curry Wheatberry Rice

Time To Prepare: ten minutes
Time to Cook: 1 hour fifteen minutes
Yield: Servings 5

Ingredients:
- ¼ cup milk
- ½ cup of rice
- 1 cup wheat berries
- 1 tablespoon curry paste
- 1 teaspoon salt
- 4 tablespoons olive oil
- 6 cups chicken stock

Directions:
1. Put wheatberries and chicken stock in the pan.
2. Close the lid and cook the mixture for an hour over the moderate heat.
3. Then put in rice, olive oil, and salt.
4. Stir thoroughly.
5. Mix up together milk and curry paste.
6. Put in the curry liquid in the rice-wheatberry mixture and stir thoroughly.
7. Boil the meal for fifteen minutes with the closed lid.
8. When the rice is cooked, all the meal is cooked.

Nutritional Info: Calories 232 ‖ Fat: fifteen ‖ Fiber: 1.4 ‖ Carbs: 23.5 ‖ Protein: 3.9

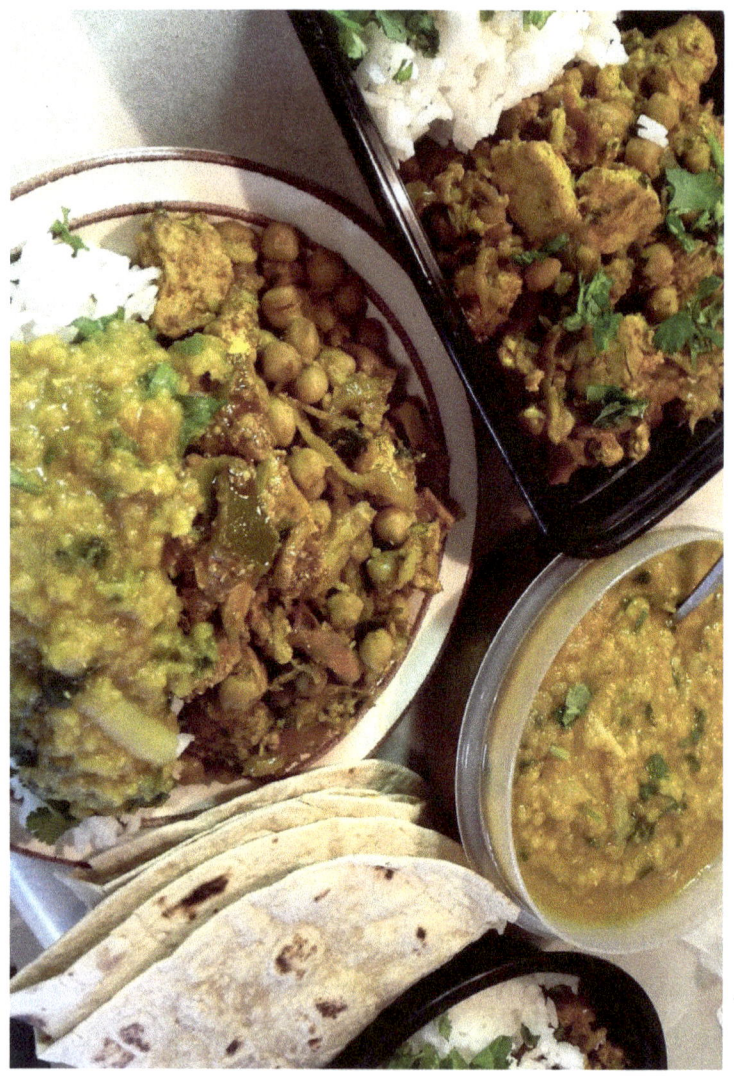

Farro Salad with Arugula

Time To Prepare: ten minutes
Time to Cook: thirty-five minutes
Yield: Servings 2

Ingredients:
- ½ cup farro
- ½ teaspoon ground black pepper
- ½ teaspoon Italian seasoning
- ½ teaspoon olive oil
- 1 ½ cup chicken stock
- 1 cucumber, chopped
- 1 tablespoon lemon juice
- 1 teaspoon salt
- 2 cups arugula, chopped

Directions:
1. Mix up together farro, salt, and chicken stock and move mixture in the pan.
2. Close the lid and boil it for a little more than half an hour.
3. In the meantime, place all rest of the ingredients in the salad container.
4. Chill the farro to the room temperature and put in it in the salad container too.
5. Mix up the salad well.

Nutritional Info: Calories 92 ‖ Fat: 2.3 ‖ Fiber: 2 ‖ Carbs: 15.6 ‖ Protein: 3.9

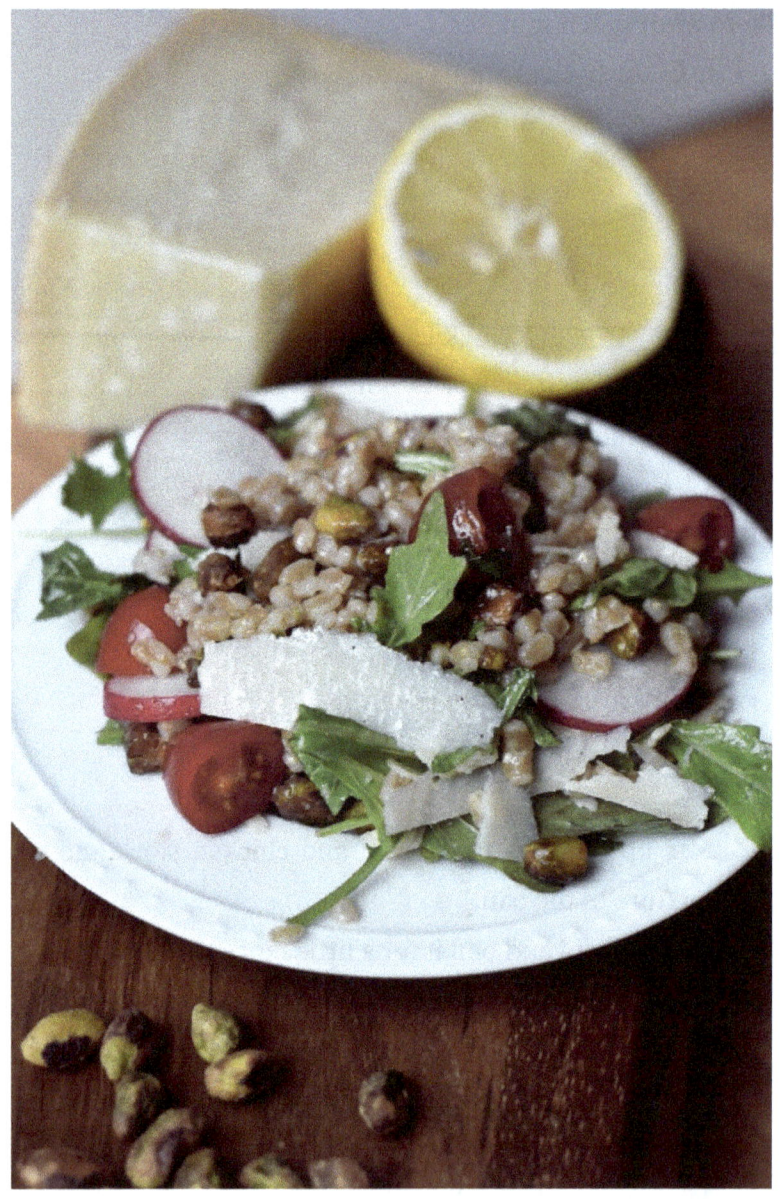

Feta Cheese Salad

Time To Prepare: ten minutes
Time to Cook: 0 minutes
Yield: Servings 2

Ingredients:
- 1 tbsp. olive oil (extra virgin)
- 1 tsp balsamic vinegar
- 2 cucumbers
- 30 g feta cheese
- 4 spring onions
- 4 tomatoes
- Salt

Directions:
1. Cube the tomatoes and cucumbers.
2. Thinly slice the onions.
3. Crush the feta cheese.
4. Mix tomatoes, onions, and cucumbers.
5. Put olive oil, vinegar, and a small amount of salt.
6. Put in feta cheese.
7. Enjoy your meal!

Nutritional Info: ‖ Calories: 221 kcal ‖ Protein: 9.24 g ‖ Fat: 13.84 g ‖ Carbohydrates: 17.18 g

Fresh Strawberry Salsa

Time To Prepare: ten minutes
Time to Cook: 0 minutes
Yield: Servings 6-8

Ingredients:

- ¼ cup fresh lime juice
- ½ cup fresh cilantro
- ½ cup red onion, finely chopped
- ½ teaspoon lime zest, grated
- 1-2 jalapeños, deseeded, finely chopped
- 2 kiwi fruit, peeled, chopped
- 2 pounds fresh ripe strawberries, hulled, chopped
- 2 teaspoons pure raw honey

Directions:

1. Put in lime juice, lime zest and honey into a big container and whisk well.
2. Put in remaining ingredients then mix thoroughly. Cover and set aside for a while for the flavors to set in and serve.

Nutritional Info: ‖ Calories: 119 kcal ‖ Protein: 9.26 g ‖ Fat: 4.38 g ‖ Carbohydrates: 11.73 g

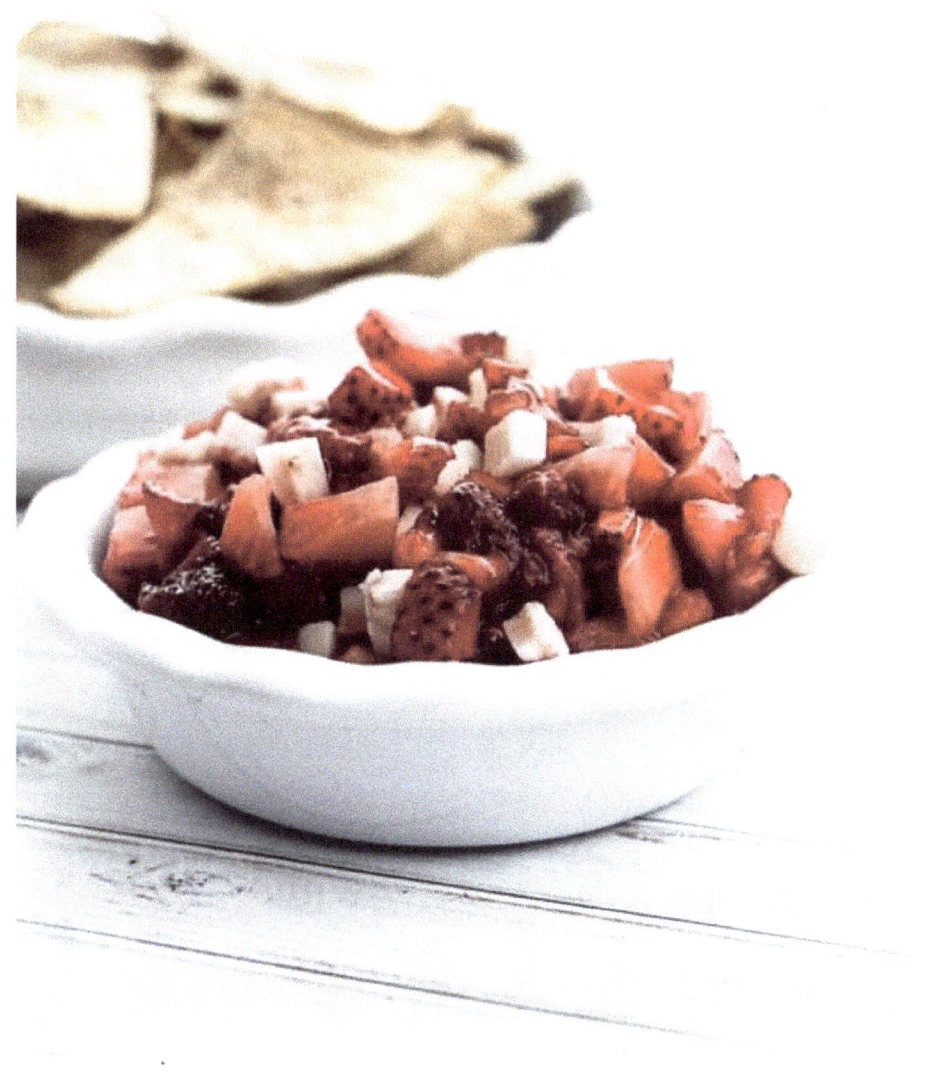

SAUCES AND DRESSINGS

Creamy Avocado Dressing

Time To Prepare: ten minutes
Time to Cook: 0 minutes
Yield: Servings 2-4

Ingredients:

- ½ cup of extra-virgin olive oil
- 1 clove of garlic, chopped
- 1 tsp of honey or maple syrup
- 2 small or 1 large-sized avocado, pitted and chopped
- 2 tsp of lemon or lime juice
- 3 tbsp. of chopped parsley
- 3 tbsp. of red wine vinegar
- Onion powder
- Some Kosher salt and ground black pepper

Directions:

1. Combine all ingredients into a blender, apart from the oil. As the ingredients are mixed, progressively put in the oil

into the mixture. Blend until the desired smoothness is achieved or becomes liquidy.
2. Use as a vegetable or fruit salad dressing. Put in your fridge for maximum 5 days.

Nutritional Info: ‖ Calories: 300 kcal ‖ Protein: 4.09 g ‖ Fat: 27.9 g ‖ Carbohydrates: 11.41 g

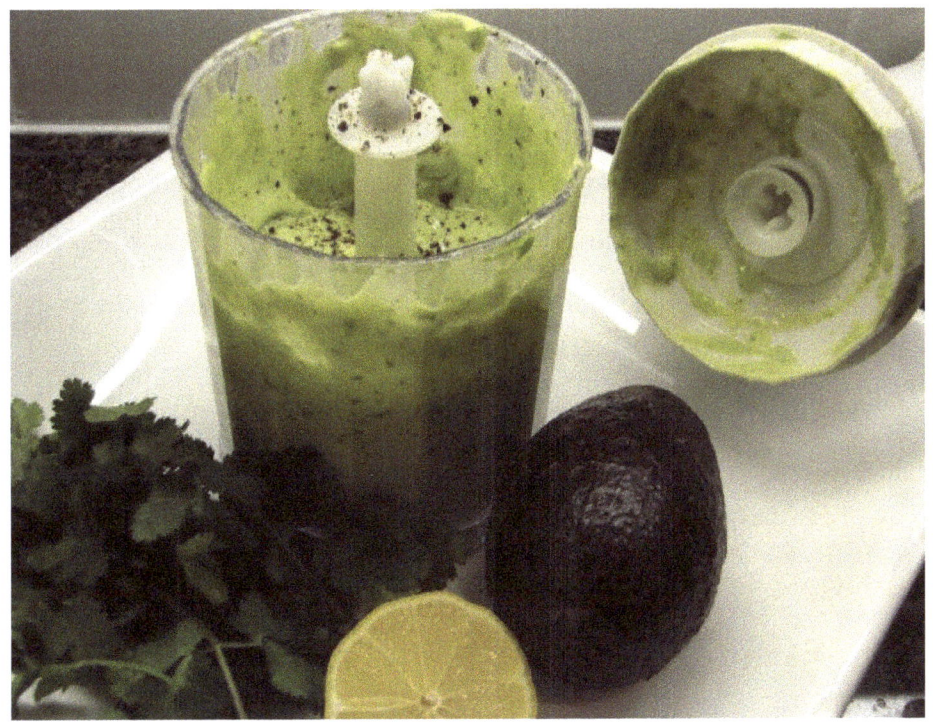

Creamy Homemade Greek Dressing

Time To Prepare: ten minutes
Time to Cook: 0 minutes
Yield: Servings 2-4

Ingredients:

- ¼ cup non-dairy milk (e.g., almond, rice milk)
- ½ cup of high-quality mayonnaise, without preservatives
- ½ tsp dried basil
- ½ tsp dried oregano
- ½ tsp parsley
- ½ tsp thyme
- 1/3 cup of extra-virgin olive oil
- 1/4 cup of white wine vinegar
- 2 cloves of garlic, minced
- 2 tbsp. of lemon or lime juice
- 2 tsp of honey
- A few tablespoons of water
- Some Kosher salt and pepper

Directions:

1. Put all together ingredients in a mason jar and shake, cover firmly, and shake thoroughly. Place in your fridge for a few

hours before you serve or serve instantly on your favorite vegetable or fruit salad.
2. Shake well before use. Put in your fridge for maximum 5 days.
3. You may put in a few tablespoons of water to tune the consistency as per your preference.

Nutritional Info: ‖ Calories: 474 kcal ‖ Protein: 2.08 g ‖ Fat: 50.1 g ‖ Carbohydrates: 5.31 g

SNACKS

Brownies Avocado

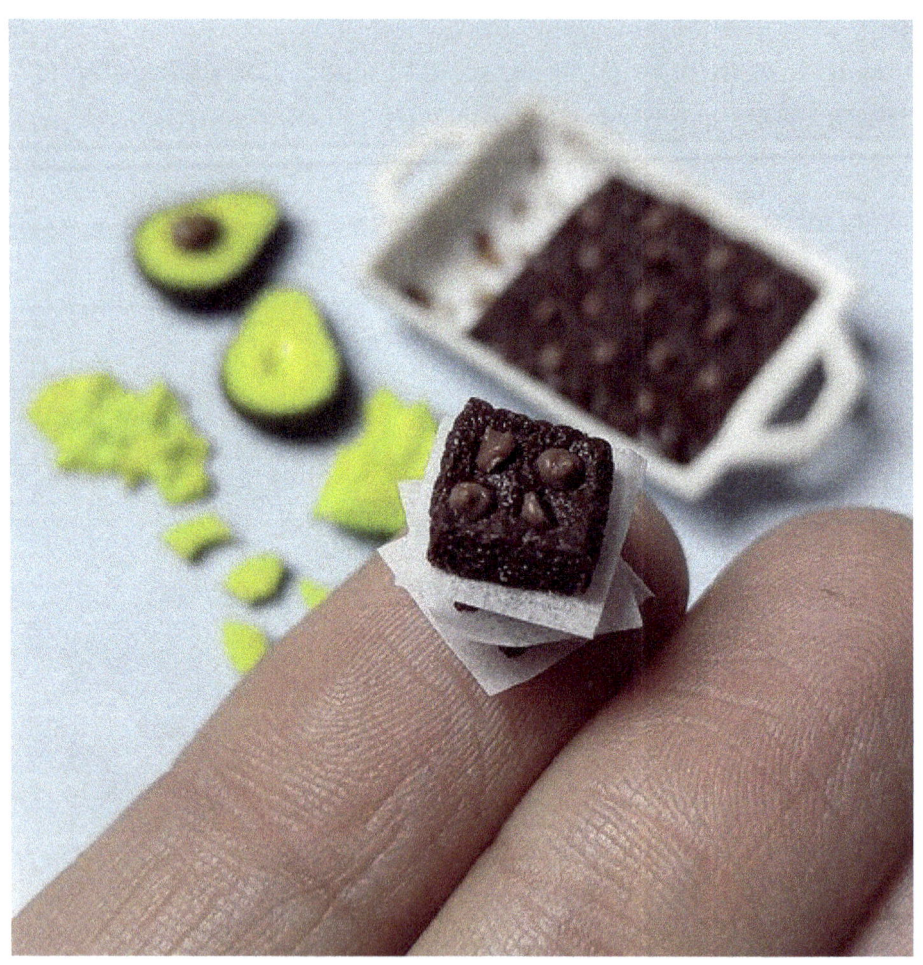

Time To Prepare: ten minutes

Time to Cook: twenty-five minutes
Yield: Servings 6-8

Ingredients:
- ½ cup almond meal
- 1 ½ teaspoon instant coffee (with or without caffeine, as you wish)
- 2 teaspoons ground cinnamon
- ½ teaspoon salt
- 2 cups nuts or seeds, chopped
- 1 avocado
- 1 apple, cored and chopped, with the skin on
- 1 cup cooked and diced sweet potato
- 4 tablespoons ground chia seeds
- 1 teaspoon vanilla
- ½ cup almond butter
- ½ cup coconut butter, softened
- 1/4 cup coconut oil
- 2 1/4 cup stevia
- 3/4 cup cocoa powder

Directions:
1. Set the oven to 350F then line a 9 by 13-inch pan with parchment. Allow it to overlap the sides to make handles for lifting the brownies out when done.
2. In a container, mix the almond meal, cocoa, coffee, cinnamon, salt, and nuts. Whisk and save for later.

3. Bring the remaining ingredients in a food processor and mix until the desired smoothness is achieved. Put in the ingredients in the container and pulse. This combination must be lumpy.
4. Pour into pan and bake for minimum twenty-five minutes.
5. Allow to cool and chill in your fridge for a couple of hours before cutting. The baked product will be a little gooey, so refrigerating it makes the brownies easier to cut. The chilled results will be fairly crumbly.

Nutritional Info: ‖ Calories: 591 kcal ‖ Protein: 11.03 g ‖ Fat: 53.8 g ‖ Carbohydrates: 26.58 g

Bruschetta

Time To Prepare: 60 minutes
Time to Cook: 0 minutes
Yield: Servings 4

Ingredients:

- ¼ cup of extra virgin olive oil
- ¼ teaspoon of ground black pepper
- 1 red onion, diced
- 1 teaspoon of sea salt
- 2 cloves of garlic, minced
- 2 tablespoons of balsamic vinegar
- 4 medium tomatoes, diced

Directions:

1. Put all together the ingredients into a big container, and stir slowly.
2. Place in your fridge for an hour before you serve on gluten-free toast (toast is not included in nutritional information)

Nutritional Info: ‖ Total Carbohydrates: 8g ‖ Fiber: 2g ‖ Net Carbohydrates: ‖ Protein: 1g ‖ Total Fat: 14g ‖ Calories: 156

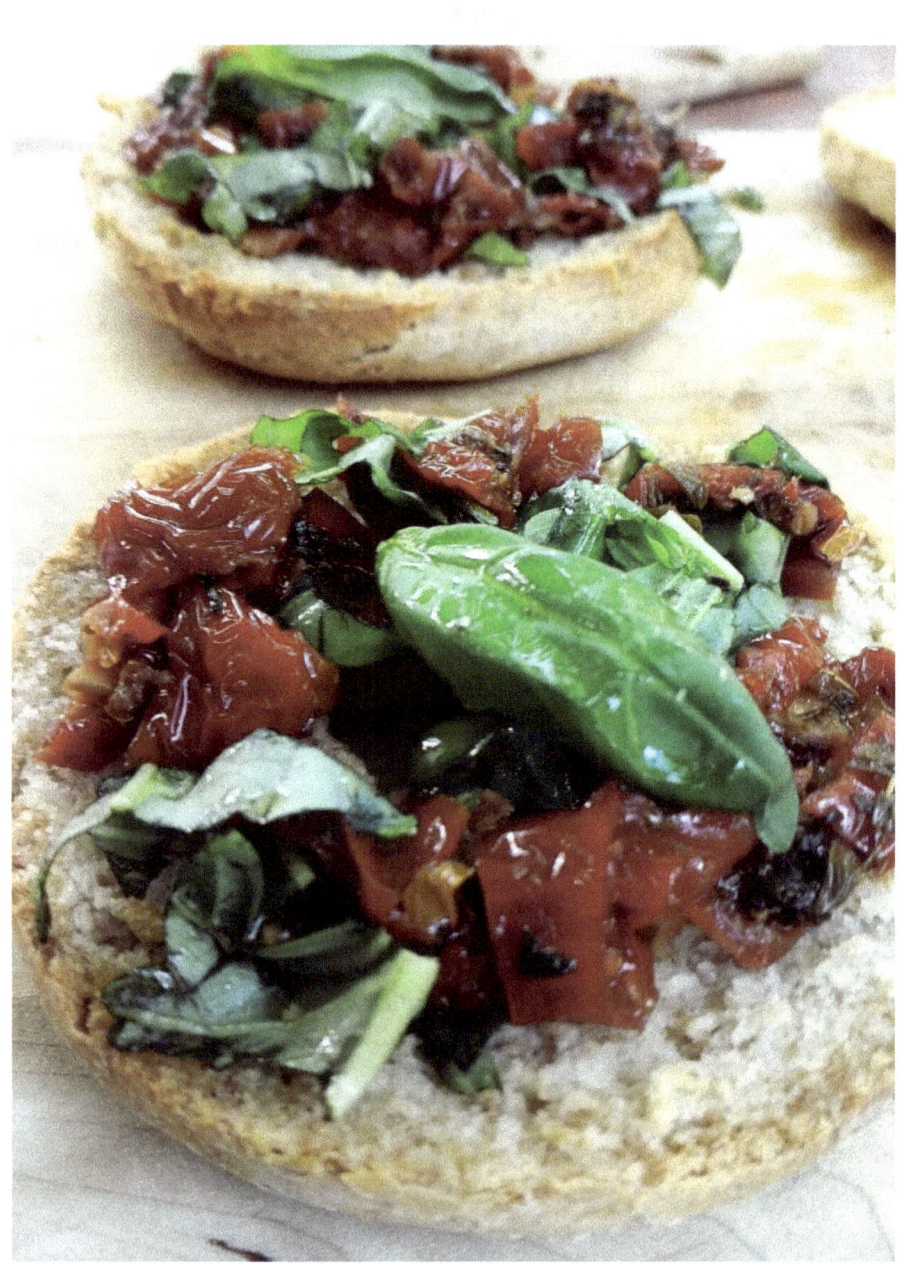

Brussels Sprout Chips

Time To Prepare: ten minutes
Time to Cook: ten minutes
Yield: Servings 4

Ingredients:

- 2 cups Brussels sprout leaves
- 2 tablespoons ghee
- Kosher salt
- Lemon zest

Directions:

1. Set the oven to 350F, then cover two cookie sheets using parchment paper.
2. Place the leaves in a huge container and pour melted ghee over the top, and put in salt.
3. Bake for minimum 8 to ten minutes or until the leaves are crunchy. If they are tender at all, put them back in your oven.
4. While still hot, drizzle the lemon zest over the leaves. Serve warm.

Nutritional Info: ‖ Calories: 42 kcal ‖ Protein: 3.13 g ‖ Fat: 1.68 g ‖ Carbohydrates: 4.77 g

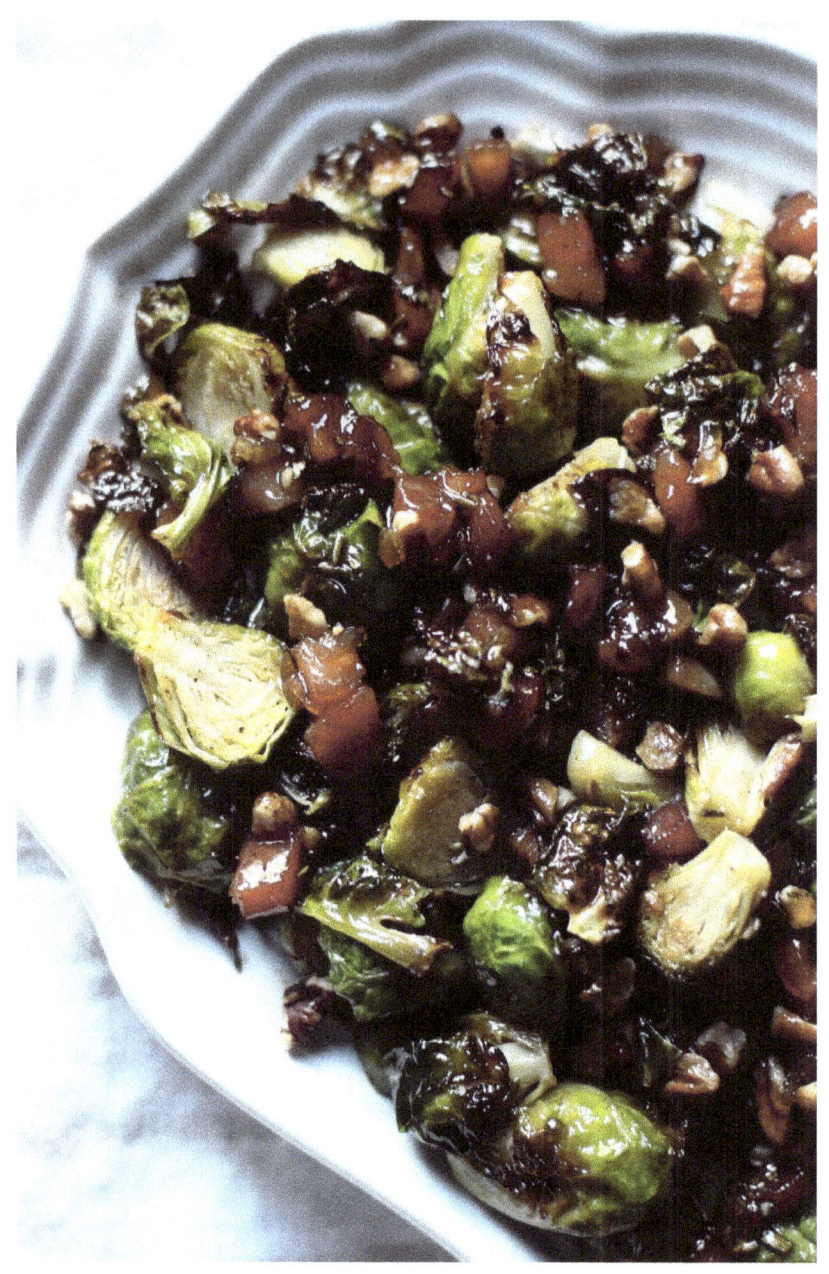

Buttered Banana Chickpea Cookies

Time To Prepare: ten minutes
Time to Cook: twelve minutes
Yield: Servings 8

Ingredients:

- ¼-tsp cinnamon
- ¼-tsp salt
- ⅓-cup chocolate chips
- ⅓-cup coconut sugar
- ½-cup creamy peanut butter
- 1-pc small banana, very ripe
- 1-tsp baking powder
- 2-Tbsps ground flaxseed
- 2-tsp vanilla extract
- fifteen-oz. chickpeas, washed and drained

Directions:

1. Preheat the oven to 350F. Grease a baking pan with cooking spray.
2. Mix in all the ingredients apart from the chocolate chips in your blender. Combine the batter for two minutes, or until turning into a smooth consistency.

3. Mix in the chocolate chips. Ladle the batter to make cookies. Put the cookies in the pan, and bake for about twelve minutes.

Nutritional Info: ‖ Calories: 372 ‖ Fat: 12.4g ‖ Protein: 18.6g ‖ Sodium: 174mg ‖ Total Carbohydrates: 58.1g ‖ Fiber: 11.6g ‖ Net Carbohydrates: 46.5g

Candied Dates

Time To Prepare: five minutes
Time to Cook: 0 minutes
Yield: Servings 2

Ingredients:
- 2 tablespoons of dark cocoa nibs
- 2 tablespoons of peanut butter
- 4 pitted Medjool dates

Directions:
1. Cut the pitted dates in half, and spread half a tablespoon of peanut butter on each date.
2. Top each date with half a tablespoon of dark cocoa nibs.
3. Split the candied dates between two plates, and enjoy!

Nutritional Info: ‖ Total Carbohydrates: 20g ‖ Fiber: 3g ‖ Net Carbohydrates: ‖ Protein: 5g ‖ Total Fat: 12g ‖ Calories: 187

Carrot Sticks with Avocado Dip

Time To Prepare: ten minutes
Time to Cook: 0 minutes
Yield: Servings 6

Ingredients:

- ½ cup cilantro, firmly packed
- ½ onion
- 1 big avocado, pitted
- 1 tablespoon of chili-garlic sauce or chili sauce
- 2 tablespoon olive oil
- 6 ounces shelled edamame
- Juice of one lemon
- Salt and pepper

Directions:

1. Put the edamame, cilantro, onion, and chili sauce in a blender or food processor. Pulse it to cut and mix the ingredients. Put in the avocado and the lemon juice. Slowly put in the olive oil as you blend. Move to a jar.
2. Scoop 2 spoons and serve with carrot sticks.

Nutritional Info: ‖ Calories: 154 kcal ‖ Protein: 5.16 g ‖ Fat: 11.96 g ‖ Carbohydrates: 8.44 g

Cashew "Humus"

Time To Prepare: ten minutes
Time to Cook: 0 minutes
Yield: Servings 1

Ingredients:

- ¼ Cup Water
- ¼ Teaspoon Sea Salt, Fine
- ½ Teaspoon Ground Ginger
- 1 Cup Cashews, Raw & Soaked in Water for fifteen Minutes & Drained
- 1 Tablespoon Olive Oil
- 1 Teaspoon Lemon juice, Fresh
- 2 Cloves Garlic
- 2 Teaspoon Coconut Aminos
- Pinch Cayenne Pepper

Directions:

1. Blend all ingredients together, and ensure to scrape the sides.
2. Continue to combine until the desired smoothness is achieved, and then place in your fridge it before you serve.

Nutritional Info: ‖ Calories: 112 ‖ Protein: 2.9 Grams ‖ Fat: 8.8 Grams ‖ Carbohydrates: 5.3 Grams

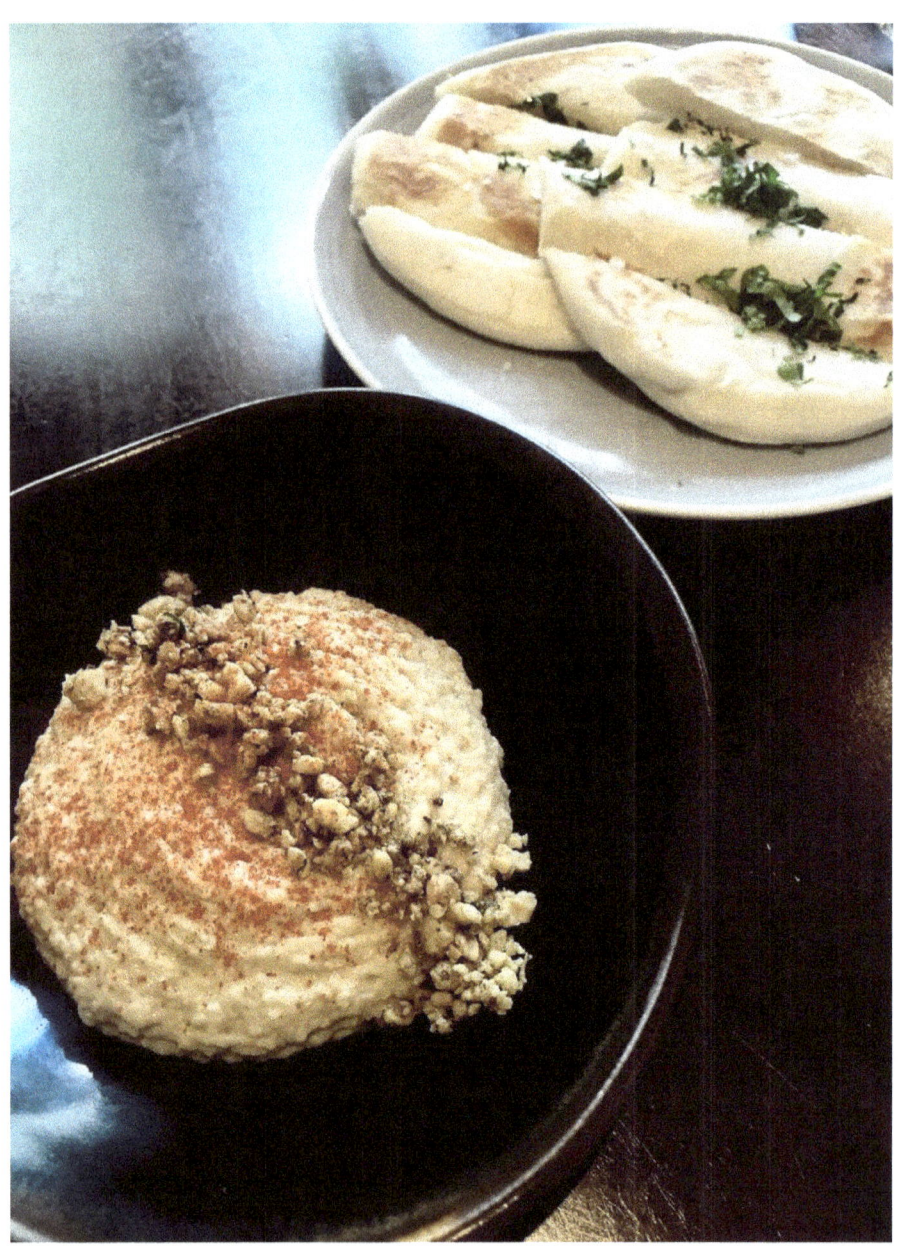

SOUPS AND STEWS

Chicken Chili Blanco

Time To Prepare: ten minutes
Time to Cook: twenty minutes
Yield: Servings 4

Ingredients:

- ¼ teaspoon cayenne pepper
- 1 tablespoon ghee
- 1 teaspoon chili powder
- 2 (4-ounce) cans diced mild green chiles with their liquid
- 2 scallions, cut
- 2 small onions, chopped
- 2 teaspoons dried oregano
- 4 cups chicken broth or vegetable broth
- 4 cups shredded cooked chicken
- 4 cups white beans, drained and washed well
- 4 teaspoons ground cumin
- 6 garlic cloves, minced

Directions:

1. In a huge soup pot on moderate heat, melt the ghee.

2. Put in the onions and garlic, and sauté for five minutes.
3. Place the chiles, and cook for a couple of minutes, stirring.
4. Mix in the beans, broth, cumin, oregano, chili powder, and cayenne pepper. Heat it until it simmers.
5. Put in the chicken, bring to a simmer, decrease the heat to moderate-low, and cook for about ten minutes. Serve instantly, sprinkled with the scallions.

Nutritional Info: Calories: 304 ‖ Total Fat: 4g ‖ Saturated Fat: 2g ‖ Cholesterol: 0mg ‖ Carbohydrates: 46g ‖ Fiber: 12g ‖ Protein: 21g

Chicken Tortilla Soup

Time To Prepare: ten minutes
Time to Cook: twenty minutes
Yield: Servings 8-10

Ingredients:

- 1 teaspoon cayenne pepper or to taste
- 2 cups onions, chopped
- 2 teaspoons chili powder
- 2 teaspoons cumin powder
- 2 teaspoons dried oregano
- 2 teaspoons garlic powder
- 4 cups carrots, cut
- 4 cups celery, cut
- 4 cups water
- 4 teaspoons olive oil
- 6 cups rotisserie chicken, skinless, chopped or shredded
- 8 cloves garlic, minced
- 8 cups chicken broth
- 8 medium tomatoes, chopped
- Avocado, peeled, pitted, chopped
- For the topping: Use any (not necessary)
- Fresh cilantro, chopped
- Greek yogurt
- Pepper powder to taste

- Salt to taste
- Tortilla chips, crumbled

Directions:
1. Put a soup pot on moderate heat. Put in oil.
2. When the oil is warmed, put the onion and celery and sauté until slightly soft.
3. Put in garlic and sauté for a few seconds until aromatic. Stir in the tomatoes and cook until tender. Remove the heat.
4. Move into a blender. Put in water and blend until the desired smoothness is achieved.
5. Put back the mixed mixture into the pot. Put in the remaining ingredients and stir.
6. If it's beginning to boil, reduce the heat then simmer until vegetables are tender.
7. Ladle into soup bowls before you serve.

Nutritional Info: Calories: 1593 kcal ‖ Protein: 147.22 g ‖ Fat: 102.27 g ‖ Carbohydrates: 13.17 g

Chickpea Curry Soup

Time To Prepare: ten minutes
Time to Cook: twenty-five minutes
Yield: Servings 4

Ingredients:

- ¼ cup extra-virgin olive oil or coconut oil
- 1 (fifteen-ounce) can chickpeas, drained and washed
- 1 big apple, cored, peeled, and slice into ¼-inch dice
- 1 cup full-fat coconut milk
- 1 medium onion, finely chopped
- 1 teaspoon salt
- 2 garlic cloves, cut
- 2 tablespoons finely chopped fresh cilantro
- 2 teaspoons curry powder
- 3 cups peeled butternut squash cut into ½-inch dice
- 3 cups vegetable broth

Directions:

1. In a large pot, heat the oil on high heat.
2. Put in the onion and garlic and sauté until the onion starts to brown, six to eight minutes.
3. Place the apple, curry powder, and salt and sauté to toast the curry powder, one to two minutes.
4. Place the squash and broth then bring to its boiling point.

5. Reduce the heat then cook until the squash is soft about ten minutes.
6. Mix in the coconut milk.
7. Use an immersion blender to purée the soup in the pot until the desired smoothness is achieved.
8. Mix in the chickpeas and cilantro, heat through for one to two minutes, before you serve.

Nutritional Info: Calories: 469 ‖ Total Fat: 30g ‖ Total Carbohydrates: 45g ‖ Sugar: 14g ‖ Fiber: 10g ‖ Protein: 12g ‖ Sodium: 1174mg

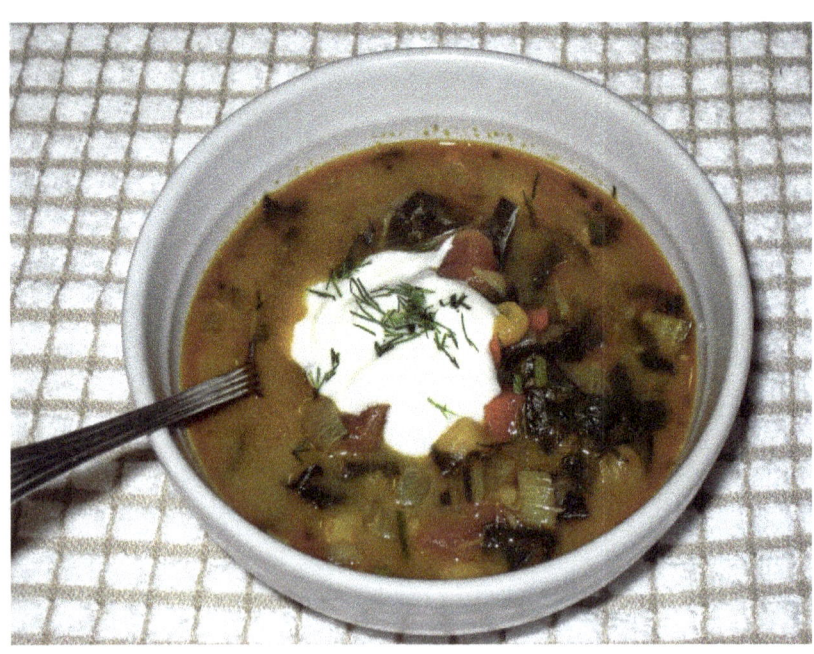

Clear Clam Chowder

Time To Prepare: ten minutes
Time to Cook: fifteen minutes
Yield: Servings 4

Ingredients:

- ¼ teaspoon freshly ground black pepper
- ½ teaspoon dried thyme
- ½ teaspoon salt
- 1 (10-ounce) can clams
- 1 (8-ounce) bottle clam juice
- 1 small red onion, cut into ¼-inch dice
- 2 celery stalks, thinly cut
- 2 cups vegetable broth
- 2 garlic cloves, cut
- 2 medium carrots, cut into ½-inch pieces
- 2 tablespoons unsalted butter

Directions:

1. In a large pot, melt the butter on high heat.
2. Put in the carrots, celery, onion, and garlic and sauté until slightly softened two to three minutes.
3. Pour the broth and clam juice, then bring it to its boiling point.
4. Reduce the heat and cook until the carrots are soft, three to five minutes.

5. Mix in the clams and their juices, thyme, salt, and pepper, heat through for two to three minutes, before you serve.

Nutritional Info: Calories: 156 ‖ Total Fat: 7g ‖ Total Carbohydrates: 7g ‖ Sugar: 3g ‖ Fiber: 1g ‖ Protein: 14g ‖ Sodium: 981mg

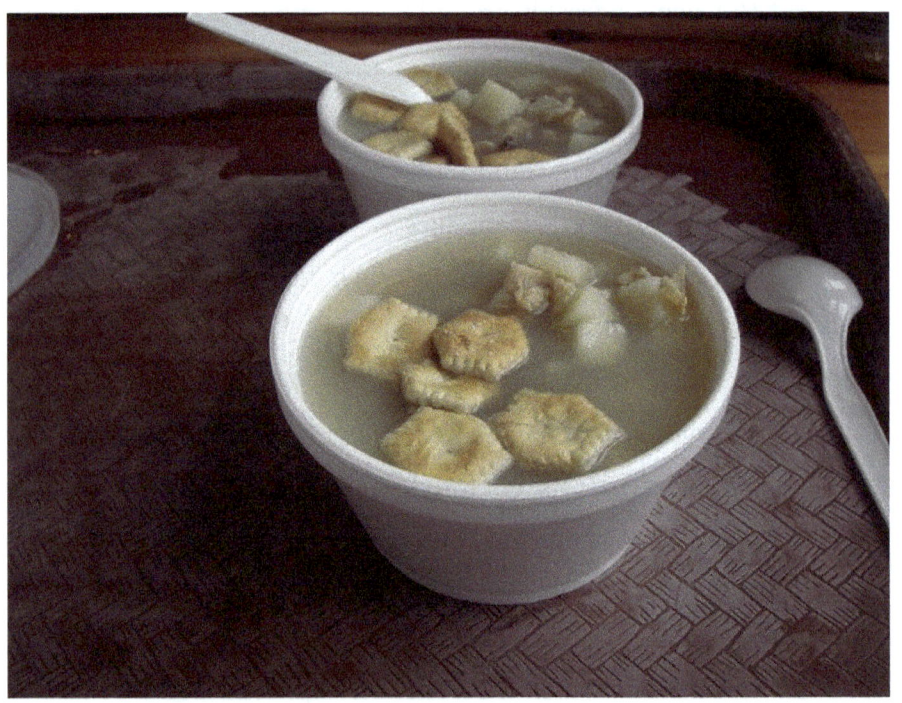

Coconut Cashew Soup with Butternut Squash

Time To Prepare: ten minutes
Time to Cook: twenty minutes
Yield: Servings 6

Ingredients:

- ½ tsp. salt
- ¾ cup toasted cashews
- 1 (14-ounce) can full-fat coconut milk
- 1 cup mung bean sprouts
- 1 small butternut squash, halved, diced
- 1 small Napa cabbage, shredded
- 1 white onion, diced
- 1½ tbsp. Ginger, peeled and minced
- 2 carrots, chopped
- 2 cups green beans, trimmed
- 2 red chili peppers, seeded and diced
- 2 tbsp. coconut oil
- 3 cups vegetable broth
- 3 garlic cloves, peeled and minced
- 4 tablespoons toasted coconut shavings
- Freshly ground black pepper

Directions:
1. In a huge soup pot on moderate heat, melt the coconut oil.
2. Place the cashews and sauté for a couple of minutes. Take off from the pan and save for later.
3. Place the peppers, garlic, and onion, and sauté for minimum 6 minutes. Then put the ginger and carrots, and sauté for minimum 3 minutes, or until the carrots and squash start to become tender.
4. Stir in the cabbage, green beans, broth, coconut milk, and salt, flavor with pepper. Simmer for fifteen minutes. Remove the heat.
5. Mix in the bean sprouts and coconut shavings.
6. Pour into soup bowls and serve instantly.

Nutritional Info: Calories: 340 ‖ Total Fat: 25g ‖ Saturated Fat: 20g ‖ Cholesterol: 0mg ‖ Carbohydrates: 23g ‖ Fiber: 5g ‖ Protein: 7g

Coconut Curried Ban-Apple Soup

Time To Prepare: ten minutes
Time to Cook: 10-fifteen minutes
Yield: Servings 4

Ingredients:

- ¼ cup toasted coconut, for decoration
- 1 big potato 1 Granny Smith apple
- 1 celery heart
- 1 cup coconut milk
- 1 ripe banana
- 1 sweet onion
- 1 teaspoon curry powder
- 1 teaspoon salt
- 2 cups Basic Vegetable Stock or low-sodium canned vegetable stock
- 2 tablespoons chopped fresh cilantro, for decoration

Directions:

1. Place the vegetable stock in a soup pot.
2. Peel the banana and potato, cut them, and place them in the soup pot. Core the apple, cut it, and put in it to the soup pot. Cut the celery heart and onion and put in them to the soup pot.

3. Put the soup to its boiling point, then reduce the heat and simmer for ten to fifteen minutes. Put in the coconut milk, curry powder, and salt.
4. Place the hot soup in a blender and purée.
5. Serve the soup hot. Decorate using toasted coconut and cilantro.

Nutritional Info: Calories: 344 ‖ Fat: 19 g ‖ Protein: 6 g ‖ Sodium: 886 mg ‖ Fiber: 7 g ‖ Carbohydrates: 40 g

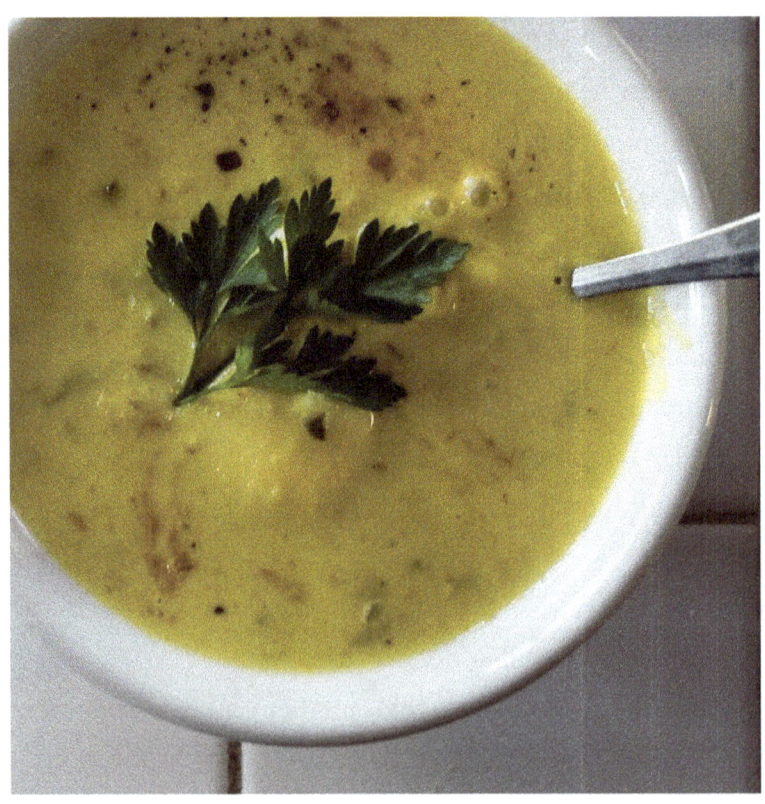

Cream of Mushroom Soup

Time To Prepare: twenty minutes
Time to Cook: thirty minutes
Yield: Servings 6

Ingredients:
- 5 cups mushrooms (cut)
- 1 tablespoon sherry
- 3 tablespoons butter
- 3 tablespoons flour
- 1 cup half-and-half
- Salt
- Ground black pepper
- 1½ cups chicken broth
- ½ cup onion (chopped)
- 1/8 teaspoon dried thyme

Directions:
1. Cook mushrooms with onion and thyme in the broth until soft.
2. Puree the mixture.
3. Whisk some flour in a pan of melted butter. Put in half-and-half, vegetable puree, and seasoning. Boil until it becomes thick.
4. Put in sherry.

Nutritional Info: Calories: 148 kcal ‖ Carbohydrates: 8.6 g ‖ Fat: 11 g ‖ Protein: 4 g

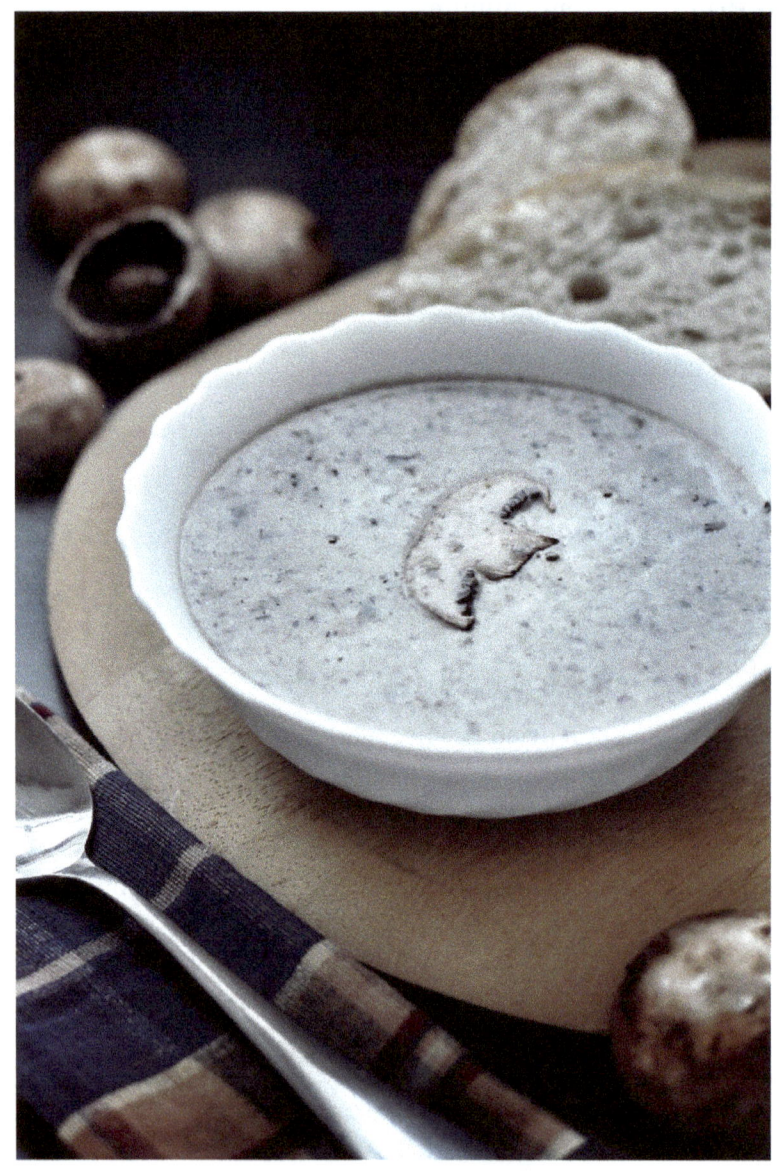

Creamy & Culture Tomato Sauce

Time To Prepare: ten minutes
Time to Cook: fifteen-twenty minutes
Yield: Servings 6

Ingredients:

- ⅛ teaspoon dried thyme
- ⅛ teaspoon freshly ground black pepper
- ¼ cup tomato paste
- ¼ teaspoon chili powder
- ½ cup plain whole-milk yogurt
- ½ teaspoon salt
- 1 small onion, chopped
- 1 tablespoon ghee
- 1 teaspoon dried basil
- 1 teaspoon dried oregano
- 2 (14-ounce) cans diced tomatoes with their juice
- 2 cups vegetable broth
- 3 garlic cloves, chopped

Directions:

1. In a huge soup pot on moderate heat, melt the ghee.
2. Place the onion and garlic, and sauté for five minutes.
3. Stir in the basil, oregano, salt, chili powder, pepper, and thyme.

4. Place the tomatoes, broth, and tomato paste, and stir until blended. Heat to a simmer, turn the heat to low, and cook for five to ten minutes. Take away the pot from the heat. With an immersion blender (or in batches in a standard blender), purée the mixture in the pot until you have the desired consistency.
5. Put in the yogurt. Blend for a minute more. Serve instantly.

Nutritional Info: Calories: 157 ‖ Total Fat: 6g ‖ Saturated Fat: 3g ‖ Cholesterol: 3mg ‖ Carbohydrates: 25g ‖ Fiber: 13g ‖ Protein: 8g

Creamy Broccoli Soup

Time To Prepare: fifteen minutes
Time to Cook: 4 hours
Yield: Servings 7

Ingredients:

- ¼ teaspoon ground black pepper
- ½ teaspoon paprika powder
- ½ teaspoon salt
- ⅔ cup heavy whipping cream
- 1 pinch cayenne pepper
- 1 red onion, roughly chopped
- 1 tablespoon olive oil
- 2 cups chicken broth
- 20 ounces (567 g) broccoli, cut into stalks and florets
- 3 garlic cloves, chopped
- 3 tablespoons butter
- ounces (99 g) Cheddar cheese, shredded

Directions:

1. Warm 1 tablespoon of butter and olive oil in a deep cooking pan, then fry the broccoli stalks and chopped onion on moderate heat for five minutes until soft.
2. Put in the garlic and keep frying for a couple of minutes until mildly browned, then drizzle with cayenne pepper,

paprika, salt, and ground black pepper. Cook for another one minutes.

3. Pour over the chicken broth. Cover the lid and leave to simmer for five minutes.
4. Take away the cooked vegetables from the deep cooking pan to a food processor and process. Lightly ladle the soup into the food processor while processing until creamy.
5. Melt the rest of the butter in the deep cooking pan, and fry the broccoli florets for five minutes until tender and soft.
6. Pour the soup from the food processor into the deep cooking pan. Blend to mix thoroughly. If the soup is too thick, you can put in some water to make it thinner.
7. Bring the soup to its boiling point, then reduce the heat and bring to a simmer using low heat for about three minutes.
8. Put in the Cheddar cheese and heavy whipping cream and cook for a couple of minutes more until the cheese melts.
9. Take away the soup from the deep cooking pan and serve warm.

Nutritional Info: calories: 266 ‖ total fat: 23g ‖ net carbs: 7g ‖ fiber: 3g ‖ protein: 8g

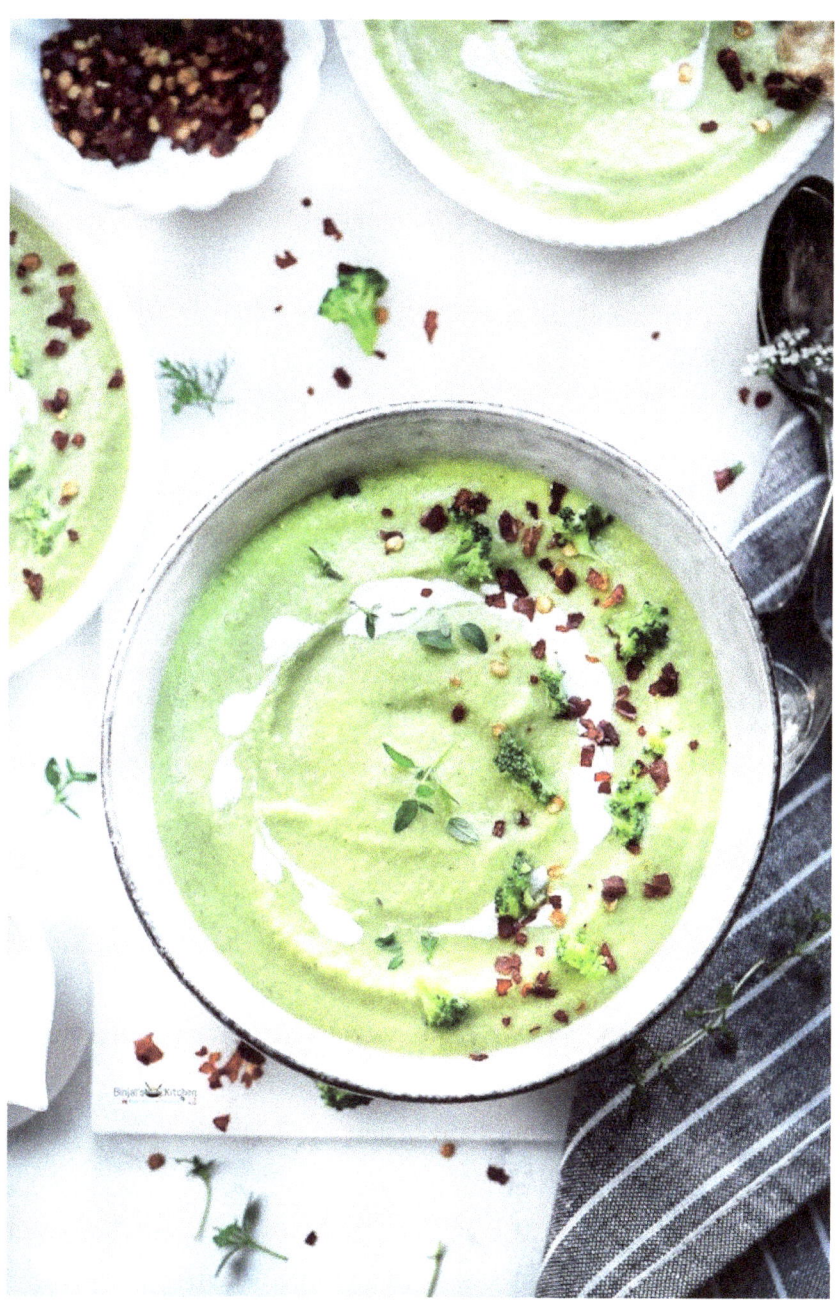

Creamy Celery And Chicken Broth

Time To Prepare: five minutes
Time to Cook: twenty minutes
Yield: Servings 4

Ingredients:

- ¼ cup celery, chopped
- ½ cup coconut cream
- 1 onion, chopped
- 2 chicken breasts, chopped
- 3 tablespoons butter
- 4 cups water
- From The Cupboard:
- Salt and freshly ground black pepper, to taste

Directions:

1. Place the butter in a deep cooking pan, and melt on moderate heat.
2. Put in and sauté the celery and onion for about three minutes or until the onion is translucent.
3. Put in the chicken, salt, black pepper, and water, and simmer for fifteen minutes. Keep stirring during the simmering.

4. Mix in the coconut cream. Pour the soup in a big container and serve warm.

Nutritional Info: calories: 398 ‖ total fat: 24.4g ‖ net carbs: 5.9g ‖ protein: 29.3g

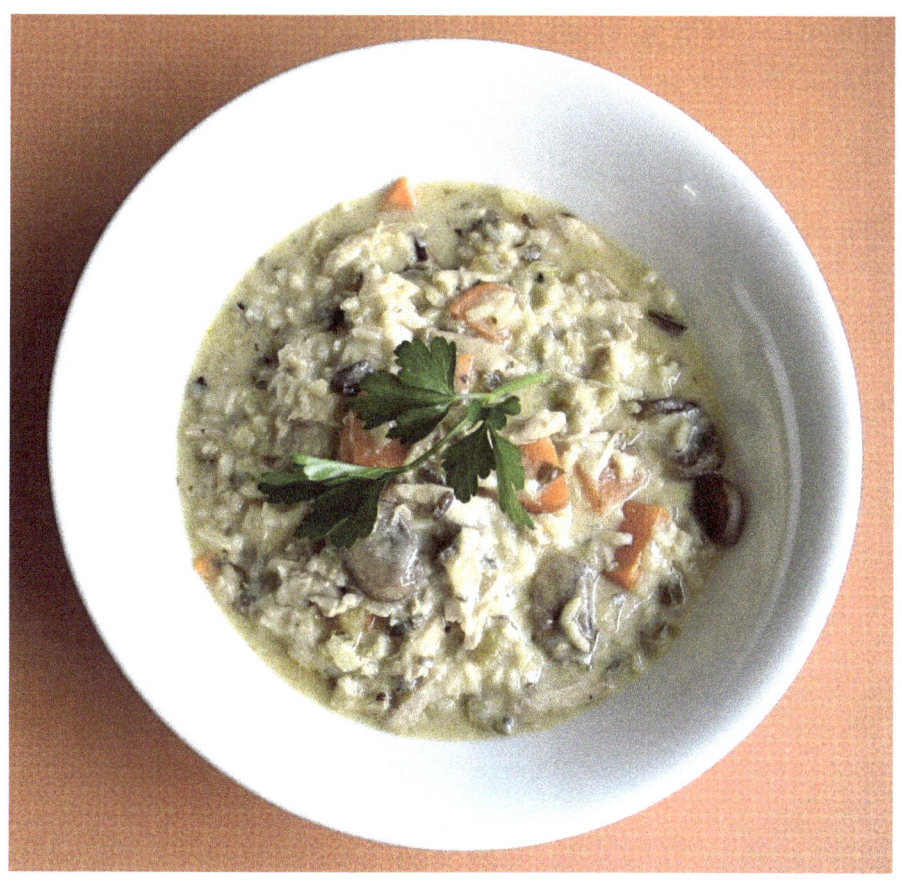

DESSERTS

Blueberry Tarts

Time To Prepare: 10 Minutes
Time to Cook: 30 Minutes
Yield: Servings 5

Ingredients:
To make the crust:
- ½ cup Raisins
- ½ tsp. Himalayan Salt
- 1 cup Cashews
- 1 cup Dates
- 1 cup Walnuts

To make the filling:
- 1 tbsp. Maple syrup
- 1/8 tsp. Cinnamon
- 4 cups Blueberries

Directions:
1. To make this yummy dessert fare, keep all the nuts in a food processor and process the nuts until it becomes coarse flour.
2. After this, spoon in the dates, salt, and raisin to the nuts mixture and process them once more.

3. Next, spread this mixture onto a greased parchment paper-lined baking sheet and place it in your fridge until set.
4. To make the filling, mix all the ingredients needed in a moderate-sized container and mix them well.
5. To finish, spoon in the filling on to the crust and spread across uniformly on all sides.
6. Top with blueberries if you wish.

Nutritional Info: ‖ Calories: 544 Kcal ‖ Protein: 12.4g ‖ Carbohydrates: 69.2g ‖ Fat:28.1g

Café-Style Fudge

Time To Prepare: ten minutes + chilling time
Time to Cook: 0 minutes
Yield: Servings 6

Ingredients:

- ½ teaspoon vanilla extract
- 1 stick butter
- 1 tablespoon instant coffee granules
- 4 tablespoons cocoa powder
- 4 tablespoons confectioners' Swerve

Directions:

1. Beat the butter and Swerve at low speed.
2. Put in in the cocoa powder, instant coffee granules, and vanilla and continue to stir until well blended.
3. Ladle the batter into a foil-lined baking sheet. Place in your fridge for two to three hours. Enjoy!

Nutritional Info: 144 Calories 15.5g ‖ Fat: 2.1g ‖ Carbs: 0.8g ‖ Protein: 1.1g Fiber

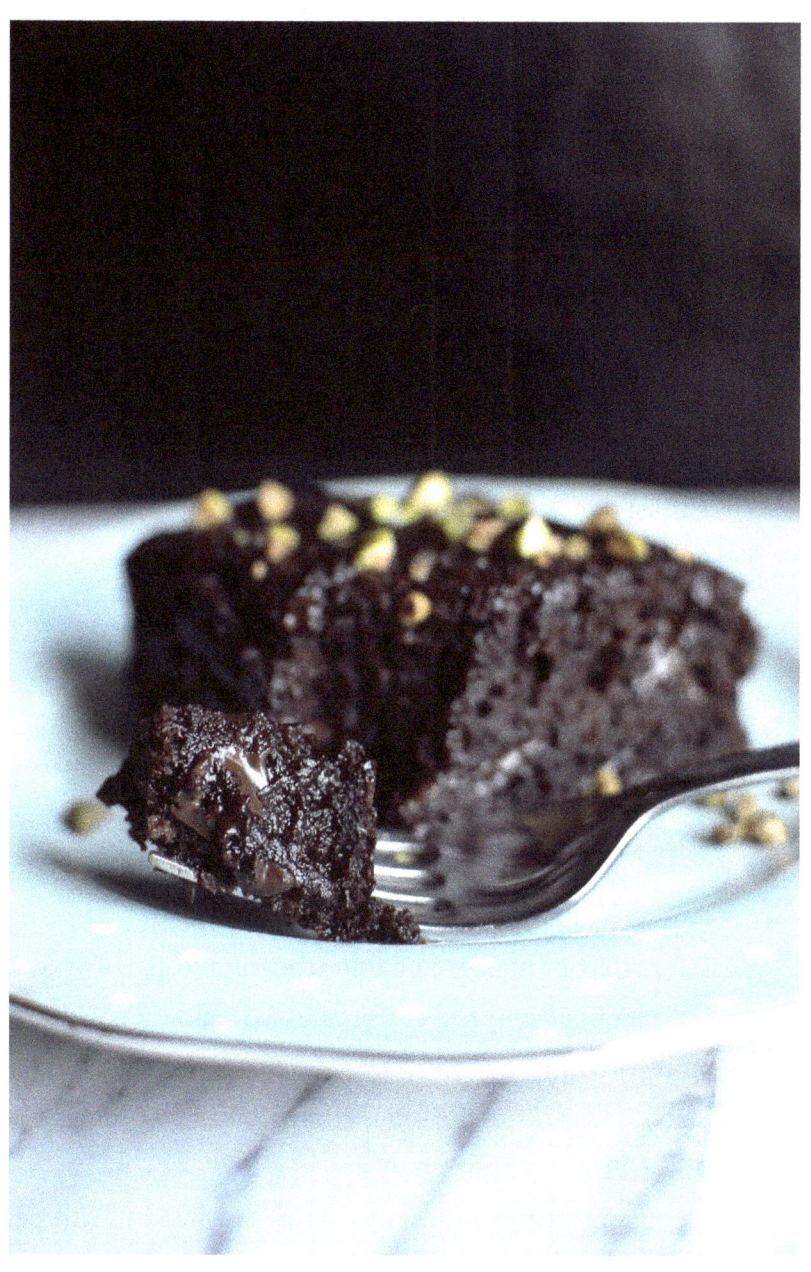

Caramelized Pears

Time To Prepare: twenty minutes

Time to Cook: five minutes

Yield: Servings 5

Ingredients:

- ¼ Cup Toasted Pecans, Chopped
- 1 Tablespoon Coconut Oil
- 1 Teaspoon Cinnamon
- 1/8 Teaspoon Sea Salt
- 2 Cups Yogurt, Plain
- 2 Tablespoon Honey, Raw
- 4 Pears, Peeled, Cored & Quartered

Directions:

1. Get out a big frying pan, and then heat the oil on moderate to high heat.
2. Put in in your honey, cinnamon, pears, and salt. Cover, and let it cook for four to five minutes. Stir once in a while, and your fruit must be soft.
3. Uncover it, and let the sauce simmer until it becomes thick. This will take a few minutes.
4. Soon your yogurt into four dessert bowls. Top with pears and pecans before you serve.

Nutritional Info: ‖ Calories: 290 ‖ Protein: 12 Grams ‖ Fat: 11 Grams ‖ Carbohydrates: 41 Grams

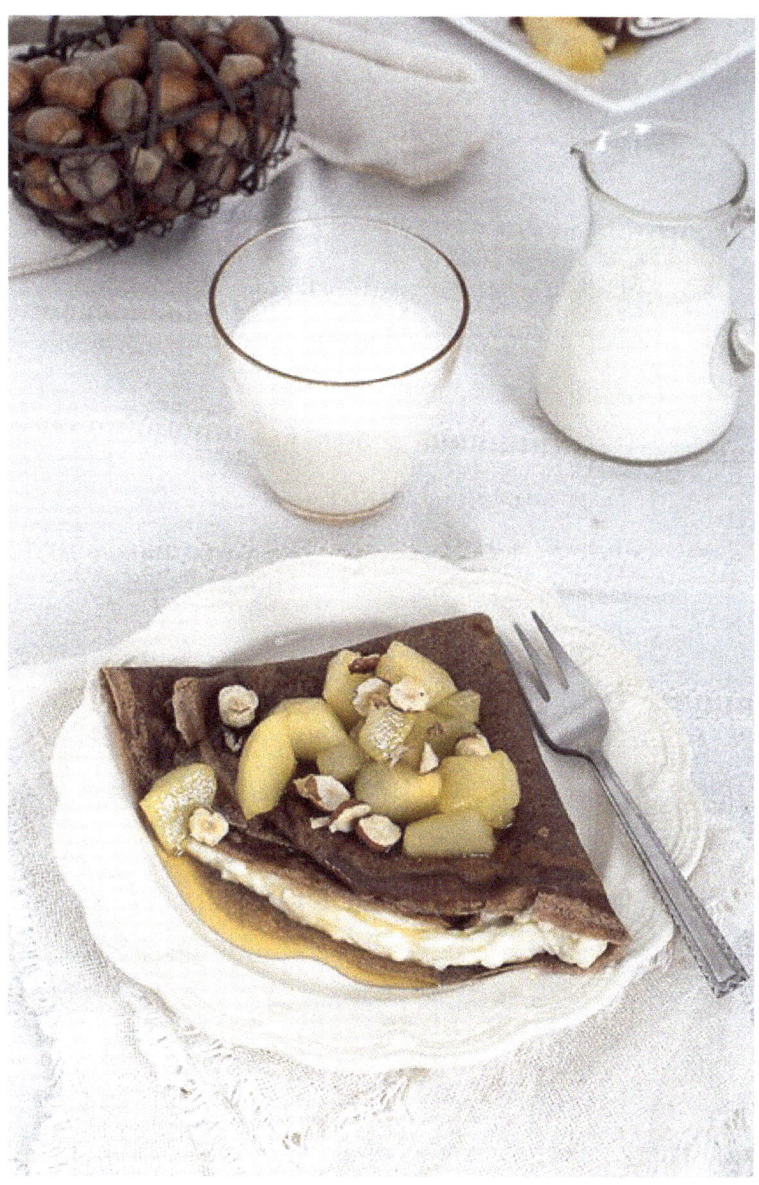

Choco Chia Cherry Cream

Time To Prepare: 4 hours and five minutes
Time to Cook: 0 minutes
Yield: Servings 4

Ingredients:

- ¼-cup chia seeds, powdered
- ½-cup cherries, pitted and cut + extra for plating
- 1½-cups almond milk
- 2-Tbsps pure maple syrup or honey
- 3-Tbsps raw cacao, powdered
- Additional toppings: extra raw cacao nibs, cherries, and 70% or higher dark chocolate shavings

Directions:

1. Mix in all the ingredients, excluding the cherries in a mason jar. Mix thoroughly until meticulously blended. Place in your fridge overnight or for 4 hours.
2. Before you serve, split the pudding equally among four serving plates. Top each plate with the cherries. Decorate using the additional toppings.

Nutritional Info: ‖ Calories: 502 ‖ Fat: 16.7g ‖ Protein: 25.1g ‖ Sodium: 68mg ‖ Total Carbohydrates: 86.3g ‖ Fiber: 23.6g ‖ Net Carbohydrates: 62.7g

Chocolate Bananas

Time To Prepare: 5 Minutes
Time to Cook: fifteen Minutes
Yield: Servings 4

Ingredients:

- 1 tbsp. Coconut Oil
- 12 oz. Dark Chocolate
- 3 Bananas, big & cut into thirds

Directions:

1. Melt the chocolate and coconut oil in a twofold boiler for three to four minutes, till you get a smooth and shiny mixture.
2. After this, keep the popsicles into the end of each of the banana by inserting it.
3. Next, immerse the chocolate into the warm chocolate mixture.
4. Shake off the surplus chocolate and put them on parchment paper.
5. Drizzle with the topping of your choice.
6. To finish, place them in the freezer for a few hours or until set.

Nutritional Info: ‖ Calories: 427Kcal ‖ Protein:5.9g ‖ Carbohydrates: 80g ‖ Fat: 15.6g

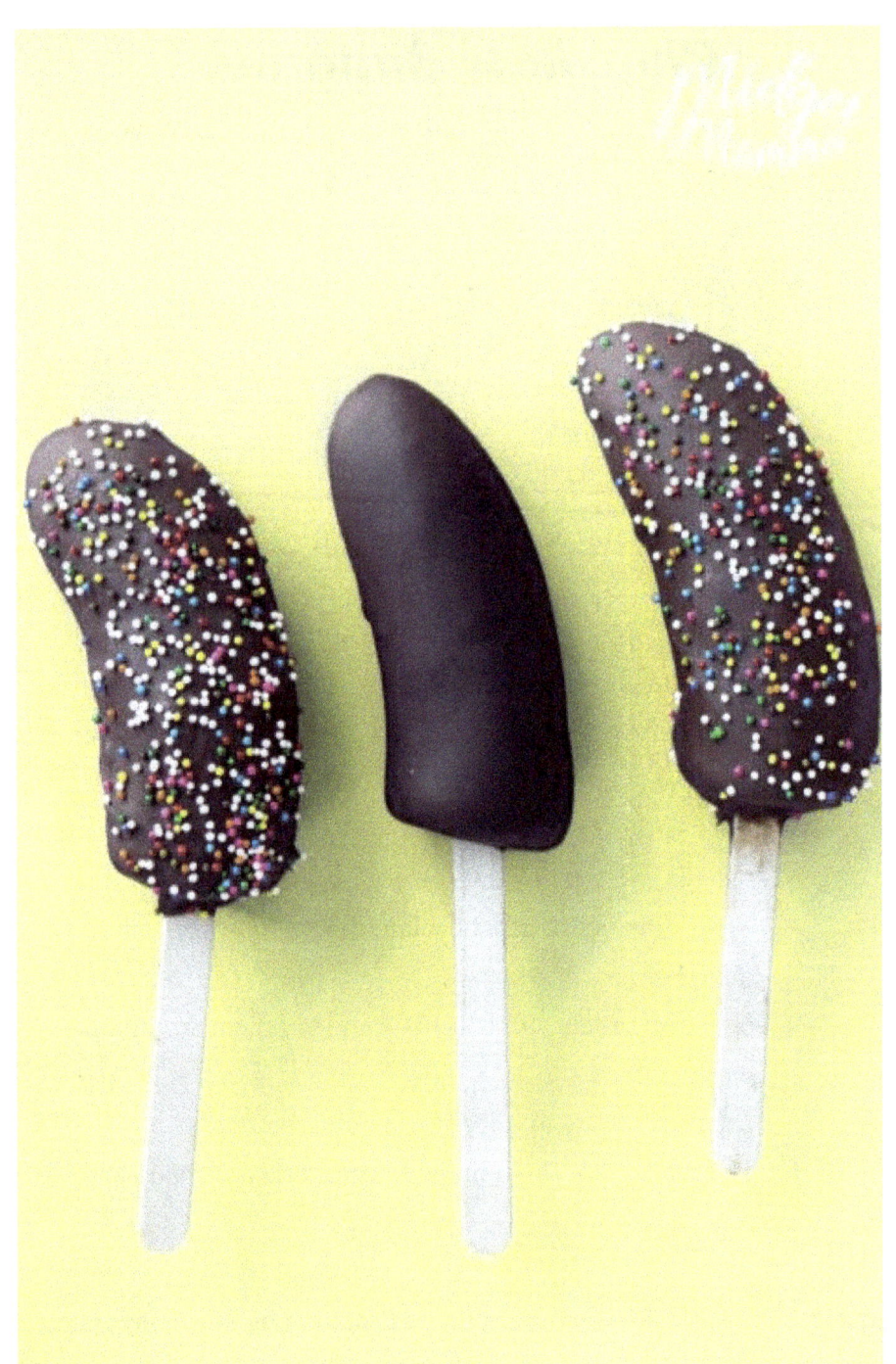

Chocolate Cherry Chia Pudding

Time To Prepare: 4 hours and five minutes
Time to Cook: 0 minutes
Yield: Servings 4
Ingredients:

- ¼ cup Chia seeds You can also use chia seed powder.
- ½ cup Sliced pitted cherries
- 1 ½ cup Any non-dairy milk like coconut or almond milk
- 3 tbsp. Maple syrup or honey
- 3 tbsp. Raw cacao powder

Additional toppings:

- Dark chocolate shavings (Preferably 70% dark chocolate or more)
- Extra cherries
- Raw cacao nibs

Directions:

1. Use a mason jar or a container. If you're using a container, just pour in the milk, maple syrup, chia seeds or powder, and raw cacao. Stir meticulously and place in your fridge for 4 hours or more.
2. If you decide to use a mason jar, just pour in the same ingredients, screw the lid on and shake vigorously!
3. Serve in separate dishes and top with any or all of the toppings I listed above.
4. Enjoy!

Nutritional Info: ‖ Calories: 811 kcal ‖ Protein: 2.38 g ‖ Fat: 83.36 g ‖ Carbohydrates: 16.88 g

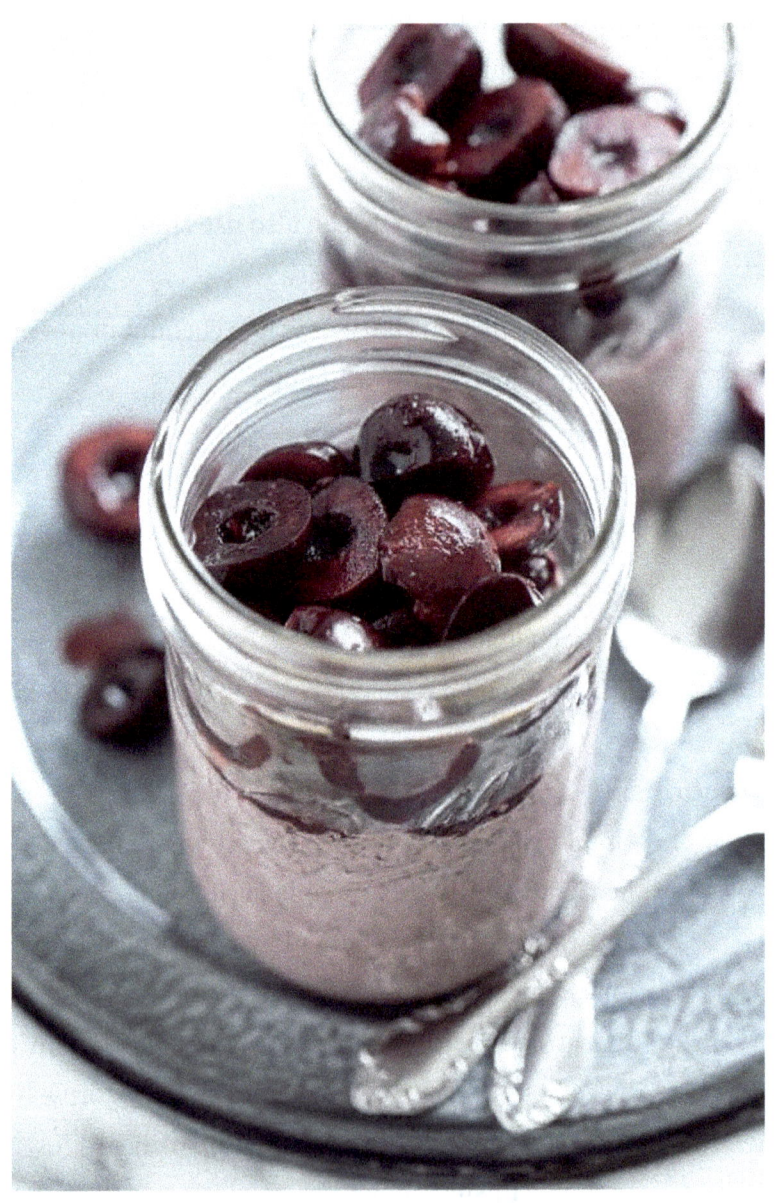

Chocolate Chip Cookies

Time To Prepare: 10 Minutes
Time to Cook: 20 Minutes
Yield: Servings 16

Ingredients:

- ½ cup Almond Butter
- ½ cup Dark Chocolate Chips, sugar-free
- ½ cup Maple Syrup
- 2 cups Almond Flour, finely sifted

Directions:

1. Preheat your oven to 350 ° F.
2. After this, mix the almond flour, almond butter, and maple syrup in a moderate-sized mixing container until combined well.
3. To this, mix in the chocolate chips and mix once more.
4. With the help of an ice cream scooper, scoop out the mixture to a greased baking sheet. Flatten the top slightly with your hand.
5. To finish, bake them for ten to twelve minutes or until they are going to get browned.

Nutritional Info: ‖ Calories: 176Kcal ‖ Protein: 5g ‖ Carbohydrates: 16g ‖ Fat: 11g

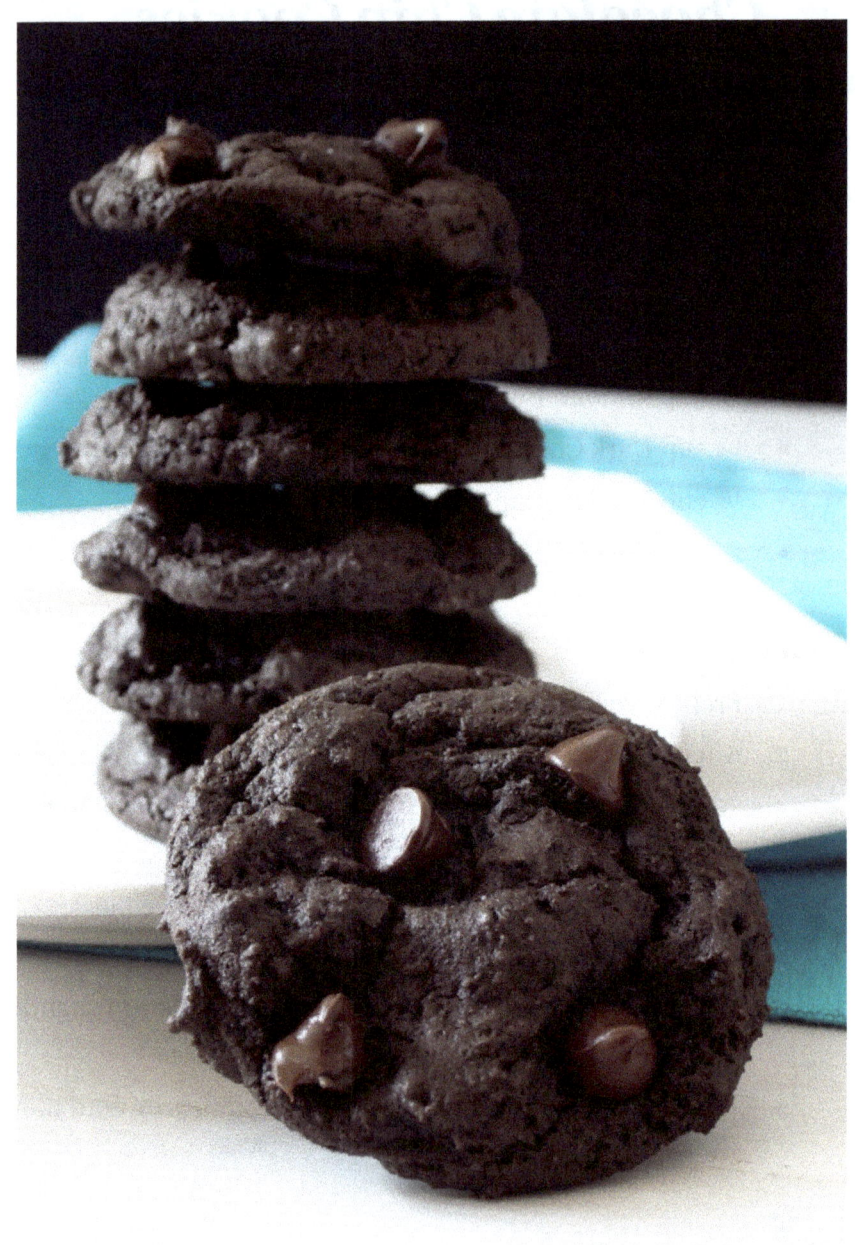

Chocolate Chip Quinoa Granola Bars

Time To Prepare: five minutes
Time to Cook: ten minutes
Yield: Servings 16

Ingredients:

- ¼ teaspoon salt
- ½ cup flax seed
- ½ cup of chia seeds
- ½ cup of chocolate chips
- ½ cup of honey
- ½ cup walnuts, chopped
- 1 cup buckwheat
- 1 cup uncooked quinoa
- 1 teaspoon of cinnamon
- 1 teaspoon of vanilla
- 2/3 cup dairy-free margarine

Directions:

1. Preheat the oven to 350 degrees F.
2. Spread the walnuts, quinoa, wheat, flax, and chia on your baking sheet.
3. Bake for about ten minutes.

4. Coat a baking dish using plastic wrap. Line with cooking spray. Keep aside.
5. Melt the margarine and honey in a saucepot.
6. Mix together the vanilla, salt, and cinnamon into the margarine mix.
7. Keep the wheat mix and quinoa in a container. Pour the margarine sauce into it.
8. Mix the mixture. Coat well. Let it cool. Mix in the chocolate chips.
9. Spread your mixture into the baking dish. Push tightly into the pan.
10. Plastic wrap. Place in your fridge overnight.
11. Cut into bars and serve.

Nutritional Info: Calories 408 ‖ Carbohydrates: 31g ‖ Fat: 28g ‖ Protein: 8g ‖ Sugar: 14g ‖ Fiber: 6g ‖ Sodium: 87mg

Chocolate Covered Strawberries

Time To Prepare: fifteen Minutes
Time to Cook: 0 Minute
Yield: Servings 24

Ingredients:

- 16 ounces milk chocolate chips
- 1-pound fresh strawberries with leaves
- 2 tablespoons shortening

Directions:

1. In a bain-marie, melt chocolate and shorter, once in a while stirring until the desired smoothness is achieved. Hold them by the toothpicks and immerse the strawberries in the chocolate mixture.
2. Put toothpicks in the top of the strawberries.
3. Turn the strawberries and put the toothpick in the Styrofoam so that the chocolate cools.

Nutritional Info: ‖ Calories: 115 Cal ‖ Fat: 12.5 g ‖ Carbohydrates: 3.2 g ‖ Protein: 6g

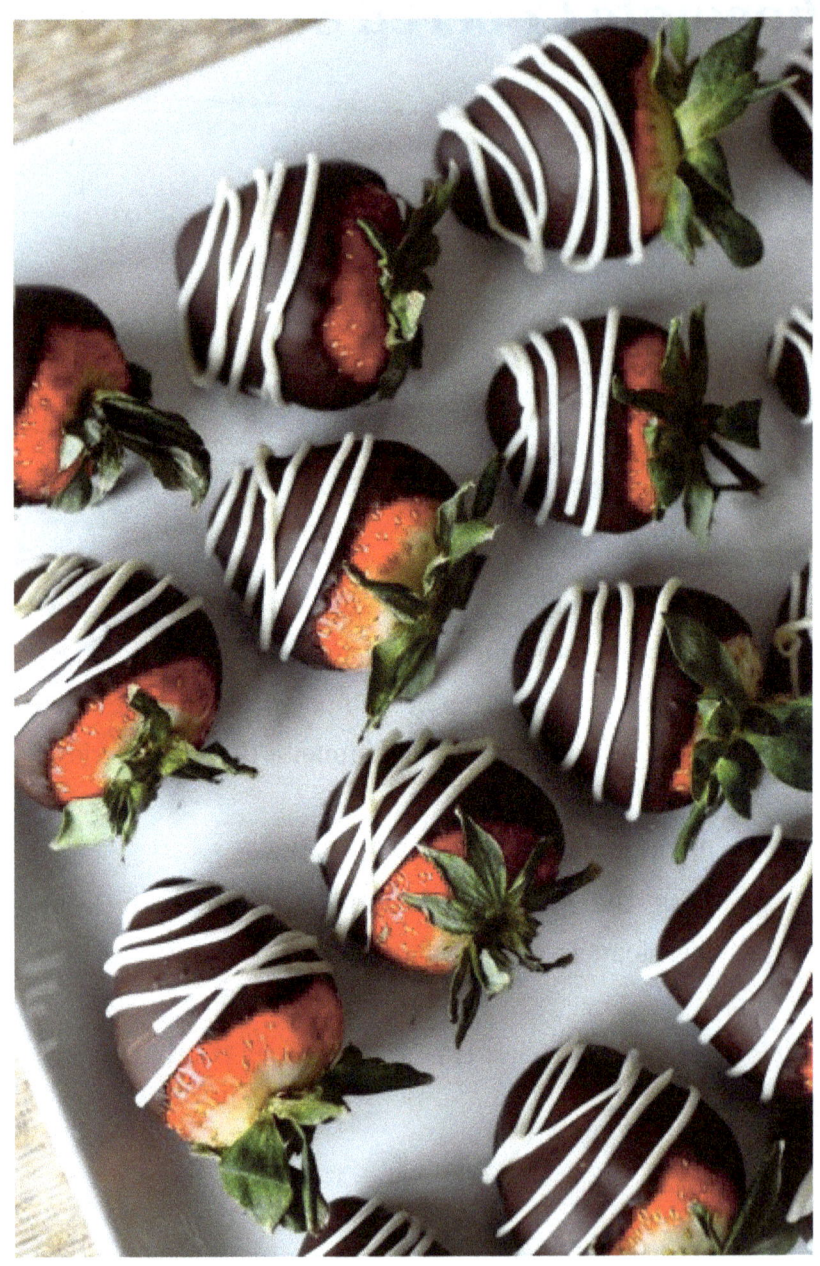

Chocolate Fudge Bites

Time To Prepare: ten minutes
Time to Cook: three minutes
Yield: Servings 10

Ingredients:

- ½ cup of coconut milk powder
- ½ cup of cold water
- ½ cup of raw cocoa powder
- 1 and a ¼ cup of boiling water
- 1 cup of coconut oil
- 1/3 cup of pure maple syrup
- 3 tablespoons of grass-fed gelatin

Directions:

1. Mix one and a quarter cup of boiling water with the gelatin, and boil for about three minutes. Next, put the gelatin mixture into a blender with the cold water and rest of the ingredients. Blend for about 2 minutes to help the gelatin solidify.
2. Put the mixture into the bottom of a greased baking dish, then place in your fridge until firm.
3. Cut into little serving squares.

Nutritional Info: ‖ Total Carbohydrates: 30g ‖ Fiber: 3g ‖ Net Carbohydrates: ‖ Protein: 2g ‖ Total Fat: 24g ‖ Calories: 317

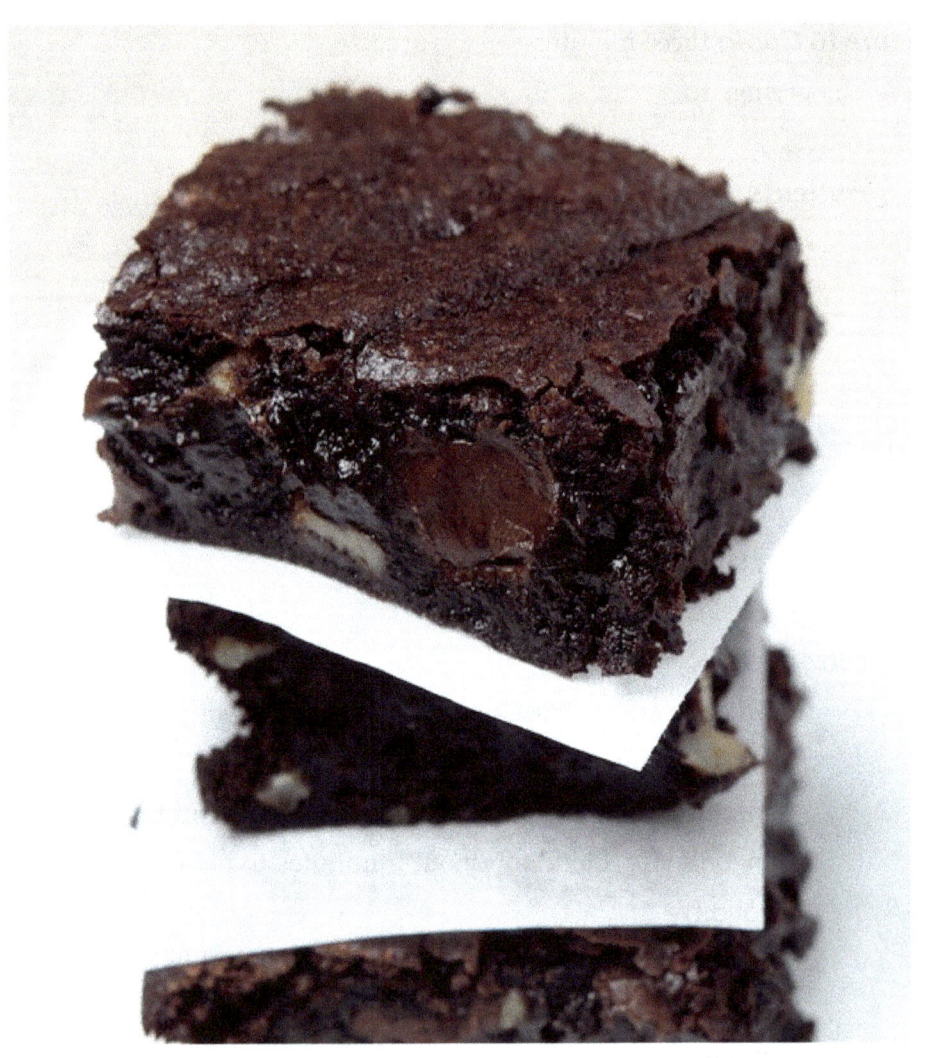

www.ingramcontent.com/pod-product-compliance
Lightning Source LLC
Chambersburg PA
CBHW070734030426
42336CB00013B/1973